MIDLIFE MINDSET

A Modern Woman's Guide To
Weathering and Prospering Through
the Stuff of Midlife and Beyond

OLGA M. TOLSCIK, MD, MPH

Praeclarus Press, LLC

www.PraeclarusPress.com

Praeclarus Press, LLC
2504 Sweetgum Lane
Amarillo, Texas 79124 USA
806-367-9950
www.PraeclarusPress.com

DISCLAIMER

The information contained in this publication is advisory only and is not intended to replace sound clinical judgment or individualized patient care. The author disclaims all warranties, whether expressed or implied, including any warranty as the quality, accuracy, safety, or suitability of this information for any particular purpose.

ISBN: 978-1-946665-37-9

©2019. Olga Tolscik. All rights reserved.

Cover Design: Ken Tackett

Developmental Editing: Kathleen Kendall-Tackett

Copyediting: Chris Tackett

Layout & Design: Nelly Murariu

Acknowledgments

To God, whose grace allows for a daily fresh start.
To my parents, Magdalena and Richard, whose
unconditional love molded me into the woman I am today.
To my sons, Adam and Alex, who bless me daily by their existence.
To my husband, Martin, who always encourages my life pursuits.

Table of Contents

Preface

This book would not exist if not for the lovely women who have graciously allowed me into their lives over the years. All of the stories you will read in this book have been fully fictionalized to provide anonymity and to allow for universalization of the feminine experience. All women, at some point in their lifecycle, will share some, if not all of these similar experiences: life, birth, loss, gain, failure, success, happiness, sadness, and everything else in between. We all need to recognize that we are all the same in one dimension: our humanity. Regardless of our age, race, religion, socioeconomic status, profession, sexual orientation, marital status, and more, we are all women, we are all human, and that is what connects us. If we can look past traditional barriers that separate us at different times—jealously, status, achievement, physical appearance, health—and focus on what makes women uniquely poised to weather the bad and still be standing when all is said and done, that truth can unify us in an unbreakable sisterhood that is uniquely our own.

I fervently hope that this book will allow us to feel more connected, supported, loved, and empowered as women, as we recognize parts of ourselves in the stories that unfold about this journey through womanhood, a true sisterhood. What women can create, let no one put asunder.

Introduction

*One should not wish anyone disagreeable conditions
of life; but for him who is involved in them by chance,
they are touchstones of characters and of the most
decisive value to man.*

GOETHE

The realization came slowly, evolving gradually over the course of caretaking. You see, my mother, my pillar of strength, rock, and best friend was leaving me. She had not decided to move to another city, nor had she and I had a massive blowout argument that ended the relationship forever. Rather, her life force was slowly dripping out of her, treatment by treatment for her illness. As a devoted daughter and a physician just like her, I felt completely overwhelmed, helpless, and, at times, hopeless. Nothing I had learned in my years of medical training could stop her continued deterioration and decline. I had no idea how I was going to keep on being there for her while tending to two young children, my private practice, my marriage, and, of course, my health and sanity.

As a psychiatrist specializing in the care of women across the lifecycle, I was doling out advice left and right to the women who were coming to see me, but I was honestly not following any of it to any consistent extent myself. I was drowning. I would often pull up to the hospital where my mom was undergoing treatment for her leukemia and lymphoma, and start sobbing in my car. This torrent of emotional release was telling me something. The question became, was I going to listen? As a typical woman, I had just slipped naturally into the multitasking, people-pleasing, caretaking role as soon as my mom was diagnosed with cancer, not giving it another thought. Accompanying my mom to nearly daily medical appointments, given her intense treatment protocol and fragile state, just became one more thing on my to-do list. It then became the top of my to-do list, with everything else being relegated to the bottom. Don't get me wrong; I would not have had it any other way. Mom's survival was my priority, and I did everything I could to support, encourage, and rally behind her. But I got lost somewhere along the way.

First, I became more irritable and impatient, and much less pleasant to be around. No one, not even my husband or children, said anything about this change, probably because they just chalked it up to the stressfulness of my mom's illness. Deep down inside, though, I knew I was not okay. My sleep, although deep because I was exhausted after long days of going non-stop, was something I craved even during the day. Sometimes, I wanted to crawl under the covers like when I was a kid and see if I could hide from everyone and everything. I think I was essentially trying to hide from adulthood, from life. My food choices were less than healthy, and mealtimes, erratic. I didn't even stop to pet our dogs, even though I know that would have probably made me feel better. I felt like a ticking time bomb.

The inspiration for this book was born from a desire to help myself and women learn to survive and thrive through the challenges often facing us in midlife and beyond. Much of what I discuss in the following chapters stems from either my personal experiences as a midlife woman or from the life journeys of friends, acquaintances, family, or the women I have been privileged to work with over the last 20 years as a physician. My inspirational mother died on February 26, 2014. I know that she would have been very proud of the changes I started to make in how I lived my life while she was ill and the life-expanding journey I have committed to since her death.

Although we typically do not welcome the struggles that that come into our lives, I have not met a woman, myself included, who has not grown emotionally or spiritually from living through a challenge. No matter what adversity we encounter along the way, I hope that you will be inspired to live by this quote from mindfulness pioneer, Jon Kabat-Zinn.

As long as you are breathing, there is more right with you than wrong with you, no matter what is wrong.

I welcome you on this journey of midlife growth and discovery. Buckle up. It's going to be a life-changing ride!

Olga Tolscik, MD, MPH

Amarillo, TX

August 2018

CHAPTER 1

Buckling In for Midlife Madness

People may call what happens at midlife "a crisis." But it's not. It's an unraveling - a time when you feel a desperate pull to live the life you want to live. Not the one you're "supposed" to live. The unraveling is a time when you are challenged by the universe to let go of who you think you are supposed to be and to embrace who you are.

BRENÉ BROWN

I think all women can agree that each stage of life has its unique challenges. For many women, the 20s may involve school or work, while the 30s may represent a time of career expansion, cementing relationships in marriage, and maybe even the diapers and sleepless nights of parenthood. I can remember exactly when it hit me that I was no longer in that age range, but rather, in midlife. After enjoying a lovely dinner with a new group of friends who were all a decade or so younger than me, the waitress had brought the check. It seemed as if on cue, the restaurant lights had romantically dimmed. As I glanced at the bill, I realized that I could not make out some of the numbers! Yikes! "Was that a 6 or an 8?" I asked myself. I tried not to make a big deal out of it, but it hit me as my younger dinner mates were already done calculating their tips and had returned to chatting merrily. I tried, as nonchalantly as possible, to pick up the check and slide it forward and back, squinting furiously at the last two numbers until I finally figured them out. Gosh, I was farsighted now, especially with the extra special light-dimming! Ugh, I thought to myself, is it already time for a pair of those plastic readers they sell at the local pharmacy? I kept this whole internal dialogue on the down low from my table companions, silently picked up my wine glass, and not missing a beat. Inside, however, my brain was screaming, "This is midlife, baby, so buckle up."

This is a light-hearted example of a midlife coming-of-age realization and not necessarily the stuff of midlife that often brings women to seek counsel in my practice.

Menopause

Let's start this exploration of common midlife issues by looking at Julie.[1] Julie, a 46-year-old woman, came in one afternoon, complaining of low mood, brain fog, weight gain, and occasional daytime hot flashes. She was in the age range of perimenopause, or menopause transition, the time that usually begins in a woman's 40s, but can occur earlier in some women. During this time, women will begin to experience various physical changes that can vary greatly in intensity and last anywhere between 4 to 8 years. One of the first symptoms that women may notice is a change in the length of time between periods, so their periods become somewhat irregular. According to NAMS, The North American Menopause Society's website www.menopause.org, menopause is defined as the final menstrual period and is usually considered to be the time after a woman has missed her period for 12 consecutive months, occurring on average around age 51.

1   All names and identifying information throughout this book have been changed to protect privacy and universalize aspects of the female experience.

Most people associate menopause with the dreaded triad of "hot flashes, night sweats, and vaginal dryness." Additionally, the hormone testosterone, although more commonly associated with men, also exists in smaller quantities in women and can also take a hit during this time, causing loss of libido, more difficulty achieving orgasm, decreased sense of wellbeing and energy, and depression. It is important also to mention that for many women, menopause can come abruptly, like after surgical removal of the ovaries, or after cancer treatments involving chemotherapy or pelvic radiation. The abruptness of this hormonal journey can often be more challenging to manage than if it occurred gradually, over a period of years. The take-home point is that each woman is unique in her experience of menopause and the key is to appreciate and attempt to manage what, if any, challenges these physical and emotional changes are affording her.

Dr. Christiane Northrup, a board-certified OB/GYN physician, has made it her mission to educate women about this unique midlife time in their health and wellness. On her website, www.drnorthrup.com, she attempts to dispel the widely held belief that menopause is strictly an "estrogen-deficiency disease," but rather, attempts to explain what is going on hormonally in midlife women in a slightly different light.

Estrogen Dominance

Dr. Northrup feels that far more women struggle during the peri-menopausal transition with the physical and emotional effects of something called "estrogen dominance." This is when hormonally, there is too much estrogen relative to progesterone in women. She believes that some women may struggle with the symptoms of estrogen dominance for 10 to 15 years. Some women have symptoms as early as age 35. So even though this is a book about midlife issues, I believe it is important that all women in their 30s and 40s understand some of the possible presentations of estrogen dominance, so they are armed with the knowledge that may help them better understand what may be going on with their bodies hormonally.

I cannot tell you how many women in their 30s and 40s feel that their health care providers have misunderstood and dismissed the symptoms Dr. Northup has listed on her website. Their providers told them that they were unlikely related to anything hormonal because they did not fit into the typically accepted age range for menopause. "You're too young" or "You just need an antidepressant," they were told time and time again, essentially deepening their sense of confusion and despair about what they were experiencing in their bodies and minds.

I hope you are sitting down while reading this because I have to warn you that Dr. Northrup's list of possible symptoms of estrogen dominance is long. Why procrastinate, ladies? Let's get to it. Possible symptoms of estrogen dominance include

- ♀ decreased sex drive,
- ♀ irregular or abnormal periods,
- ♀ water retention in the form of bloating, tender and swollen breasts,
- ♀ fibrocystic breasts,
- ♀ premenstrual headaches,
- ♀ mood lability in the form of depression or irritability,
- ♀ weight gain, especially around the abdomen and hips,
- ♀ cold hands and feet (could be related to thyroid dysfunction),
- ♀ hair loss,
- ♀ thyroid problems,
- ♀ slowed metabolism,
- ♀ brain fog and memory loss,

♀ fatigue,

♀ difficulty sleeping, and

♀ PMS.

Unfortunately for us, that's not the whole story. Dr. Northrup points out that estrogen dominance has also been linked to the following conditions: allergies, autoimmune disorders, breast cancer, uterine cancer, infertility, ovarian cysts, increased blood clotting, plus, to put a cherry on top, acceleration of the aging process. You might ask what causes estrogen dominance in some women, but not others?

When women enter perimenopause, they experience menstrual cycles where no ovulation occurs, in which case, estrogen can take the leading role in the hormonal performance, often causing the symptoms mentioned above. That, however, is not the whole picture. Other causes of estrogen dominance include excess total body fat, stress, a diet that is low in fiber, essential nutrients, and quality fats and high in refined carbohydrates, medical conditions that impair immune function, and environmental toxins.

Oh, the joys of being a woman! Now before we all get overwhelmed, it is not all doom and gloom. Passionate practitioners, like Dr. Northrup and others, encourage women to be proactive in their health to offset the impact of these symptoms and to improve quality of life.

Here are some of Dr. Northrup's recommendations to decrease estrogen dominance if you or someone you know is struggling with these symptoms.

♀ Increase nutrients in the diet by taking a high-potency multi-vitamin/mineral combination.

♀ Eat a more hormone-balancing diet with lots of fresh fruits and vegetables, adequate protein, and moderate amounts of healthy fats.

♀ Get enough fiber (through a plant-rich diet, if possible) so that it can carry excess estrogen out with each bowel movement, since if your poop sits around in your bowels for too long, estrogen gets reabsorbed instead of eliminated.

♀ Consider transdermal 2% bioidentical progesterone cream, one quarter to one-half teaspoon on your skin daily for two or three weeks before the start of your period. If your periods are irregular, Dr. Northrup recommends using the cream daily.

♀ Work on losing excess body fat and getting regular exercise. Strength training can be an especially helpful choice for midlife women.

♀ Detoxify the liver. When the liver must work hard to eliminate daily toxins like alcohol, prescription medications, caffeine, or environmental toxins, the liver's capacity to cleanse the blood of estrogen is diminished. Even though Dr. Northrup does not make specific recommendations on how to detox, many Functional Medicine practitioners can advise you how to go about doing a liver detox. Additionally, Dr. Alan Christianson, NMD, the author of *The Adrenal Reset Diet* and a naturopathic physician, offers helpful tips for naturally detoxifying the body on his website, www.drchristianson.com.

♀ Try to manage stress by regularly taking stock of the demands on your time, prioritizing and deciding which things simply must go.

Julie's Story

Now that we have had a quick lesson on how the possible hormonal changes of midlife can affect body and mind, we can now turn our attention back to Julie. After routine blood work had ruled out some other common causes of Julie's presenting symptoms, including thyroid dysfunction (more about the thyroid later), we focused on what might be going on with her hormonally. Although many women present to practitioners wanting their hormone levels checked, a single FSH (follicle-stimulating hormone) or LH (luteinizing hormone) reading can be unreliable because day-to-day hormone levels can fluctuate considerably.

In Julie's case, her hormone levels were normal. However, this did not mean that day-to-day variability in her hormone levels wasn't contributing to her presenting symptoms. Given that she was not prepared to embark upon a discussion of hormone-replacement options given a family history of breast cancer in her mother and maternal aunt, we shifted the focus on the things that we could tweak in her daily routine. We also looked at some of the stressors she was dealing with in her marriage and home life.

"I've been so tired lately." When Julie presented with those very words one day in early May, she looked like she was carrying the weight of the world on her shoulders. Besides the fatigue and the brain fog, Julie reported that she had been putting on weight over the last few years and was having difficulty getting it off. She pretty much had a running tab with Starbucks, as she frequented the drive-thru daily to boost her faltering energy levels throughout the day.

Julie had three children at home and worked fulltime as a medical biller. Her partner traveled a lot for work, so Julie was often manning the fort as the only adult, which was adding a lot of stress to her life and strain to her marriage. Once an avid swimmer in high school and college, after she got married and had children, that source of exercise and relaxation had disappeared from her to-do list. Food was a challenge, as she found herself often picking up fast food on the way home as a quicker, albeit more expensive and often less healthy way to feed her family.

The list continued, but so did our initial consultation. In our first session together, we covered everything: how many hours a night she was sleeping, how many times a day she was pooping and peeing (to look at her gut and urinary detoxification baseline), and how many times she actually scheduled herself into her daily to-do list to what were her top one or two priorities in her life. I think Julie was expecting me to give her the latest purple pill being advertised on television to cure her. She admitted that she was pleased that we were delving into so many areas in her daily life that she was slowly realizing were needing some minor, if not major, tweaking.

In Julie's particular situation, fortunately, there was nothing currently going on symptomatically that appeared to be life-threatening. We were merely putting together the pieces of her particular life puzzle. Because some parts were off, they did not fit smoothly and effortlessly together as they do when we are truer to ourselves in body and mind. We are often so distracted in our daily lives of rushing, producing, and consuming, that we do not stop and reflect on what our bodies are trying to tell us.

We tend to view symptoms that pop up as isolated annoyances that we need to eliminate in that moment. A headache, for example, is often dealt with in the most expeditious manner possible, a grope into our purse for the Advil bottle so we can get right back to the business at hand. Don't get me wrong. As a migraine sufferer since medical school, I too would reach for an Excedrin at the first sign of a migraine because I had patients to see and charts to sign off on.

Diet

After going through my own medical issues, though, I now pause and think twice before mindlessly swallowing a pill. Instead, I now do I quick mental check, like I instructed Julie to do, before rushing to medicate a symptom she was having. Let's say it's 2:30 pm and Julie's slump in energy is pushing her towards the Starbucks drive-thru yet again. I ask her to consider when she last ate, or if she even ate lunch that day. If more than three hours have passed since a meal, I recommended that she consider having a small snack like almond or sunflower seed butter on a few apple slices to regulate what might be a dip in her blood sugar level.

Hypoglycemia, a lower than normal blood sugar level, causes the brain to start to shut down, leading to symptoms like jitteriness, fatigue, irritability, anxiety, or depression that are supposed to send us a wake-up call to bring on the fuel our brains need to work properly: glucose. In addition to glucose, our brains can also use fatty acids (a.k.a., "good fats"), like those found in coconut oil or avocados, to fuel vital brain processes. When I say glucose, though, I do not mean picking up a donut to feed the brain. I am referring to a whole food like a banana and with a handful of nuts or a few baby carrots with some guacamole. I cannot tell you how many women skip meals to save calories or complain that they do not have 10 minutes in their entire workday to take care of their most vital piece of technology: their bodies. I often think we treat our cell phones with more respect than our bodies. When was the last time one of us left home without grabbing our phones? Why is it so foreign to also make it a priority to grab a few nuts or a piece of fruit to fuel our glucose slumps throughout the day? These were some of the basics Julie and I considered when we looked into possible underlying causes of her fatigue.

As our work together advanced, we continued to delve further into other potential causes for her symptoms. As her internist had already checked the basics and all appeared relatively normal, I knew we had to dig deeper and also to cast a wider lifestyle net. From a mental health point of view, Julie said that the fatigue sometimes made her feel sad that she was not feeling well, physically, but she did not have other symptoms typically associated with depression like hopelessness, changes in appetite, or thoughts of self-harm. Although she admitted that marital strain, work demands, and care for her children caused her to feel stressed, she denied feeling excessively anxious.

After exploring the possibility that subtle drops of blood sugar throughout the day might be contributing to her early- and late-afternoon energy slumps, we looked at her daily fluid intake. Although she religiously drank her coffee, she did not give much thought to drinking more water throughout the day. We talked about the fact that since our bodies are 50% to 65% water, that even mild dehydration can give certain people trouble with energy. I urged her to bring a container of water with her to work and to drink about a cup per hour. The general rule of thumb I follow is to try to drink about half of one's body weight in ounces of water throughout the day. For example, since Julie was about 160 pounds, I asked her to drink about 80 ounces of water per day or about ten 8 oz. glasses. The most common complaint I hear when I ask women to do this is that they don't have time to go to the bathroom that many times a day. Duly noted, but it's still a small price to pay to feel better naturally. So be free and pee!

After discussing what Julie should be looking for regarding pee color to informally assess hydration status (yes, I ask patients to turn around and look at her pee and poop after each bathroom visit) with light straw-colored pee being the goal. An initial goal was to improve her sluggish, constipated bowel elimination. Her normal pattern was every three days. Most people look at me as if I am crazy when, as a psychiatrist, I ask them what they are eating, drinking, and how many times they are peeing and pooping each day. Psychiatrists are supposed to focus on the brain, not the bowels, right? Wrong. Establishing proper gut health can be a powerful ally in helping women overcome depression, anxiety, and other mental health troubles.

Gut Health

There is a growing body of scientific literature that supports the existence of a direct link between the gut and brain system. In essence, if we neglect the gut, we are neglecting the brain, and if we neglect the brain, the powerhouse that makes life worth living, then we are making ourselves vulnerable to illness. When I became aware of this information, I vowed to make a discussion of nutrition and gut health a part of every patient interview. I discovered through my immune system deregulation that I needed to also work on healing my gut, to allow my immune system to get back to doing what it wants to do in the first place; heal the body.

In the last few years, much has been written about the influence of gut health on myriad mental and physical ailments plaguing women and sending them to the doctor's office for help. When you break it down to the simplest term, I think of what goes on in our stomach, and small and large intestines as critical components of our immunity and eventual healing from many of the most common complaints facing midlife women: fatigue, brain fog, constipation, low mood, and chronic anxiety. I repeat that in Julie's situation, we were dealing with a constellation of bothersome symptoms that, over time, were slowly robbing her of her energy, vitality, and overall enthusiasm for life. Julie could honestly not remember a time in the last few years that she felt joyful, excited, or motivated to do much more than survive her daily to-do list. I knew there was so much more to Julie than that and I vowed that we would keep plugging along together, putting the missing pieces of her health and vitality puzzle back together again.

For the gut piece, it came down to what Julie was and wasn't consuming. While most of us have seen commercials on TV advertising probiotic supplements, those little capsules containing billions of "healthy" bacteria, many of us still don't fully understand what introducing these helpful organisms can do for our physical and mental health. We all have billions of bacteria in our gut. Many of us forget that when we take antibiotics for sinus and other infections, we are not only wiping out the bacteria that made us sick, but all of the normal bacterial flora in our gut gets knocked out in the process. It takes time for the normal bacterial flora to get reestablished and that time frame of being unprotected can make us vulnerable to a host of issues such as superinfections or antibiotic side effects, like diarrhea. Ideally, when given a prescription for an antibiotic, we should also start taking a good probiotic right alongside it, to give our bodies the tools it needs to stay healthy.

If taking supplements is not your thing, like it was in Julie's case, there are other ways to help your gut get or stay healthy. Prebiotics are foods like bananas and sweet potatoes that, when eaten, get broken down in the large intestine and converted into "good" bacteria. Additionally, fermented foods and beverages like sauerkraut, pickles, kefir, fermented milk, or kombucha, a lightly fermented tea with live bacterial cultures are all ways to introduce some health-promoting good bacteria into your diet. I recommend going very slowly, however, by adding probiotic supplements or foods into your diet. Starting out with one capsule every other day initially, or with a tablespoon or two of sauerkraut three times a week will allow your gastrointestinal time to adjust to the introduction of new bacterial friends and will avoid the common problem of gassiness that most of us would rather avoid.

Another powerful resource for women wanting to use food as a body healing tool is Magdalena Wszelaki's book *Cooking for Hormone Balance.* Magdalena is a nutrition health coach with a passion for helping women restore balance naturally through foods healing issues from thyroid and adrenal imbalances to estrogen dominance and perimenopausal symptoms. Her website is www.hormonesbalance.com. She offers many helpful strategies that allow women to feel better by tweaking their daily eating routine to improve energy and restore vitality. Although Julie couldn't tell me that helping heal her gut had completely cured her fatigue, she was happy to report that she was much more regular with her bowel movements for the first time in her adult life. She was able to do that without taking stool softeners or laxatives. She was motivated to keep exploring ways to heal her body through nutrition. I still call that a win-win situation.

In addition to the probiotics, Julie and I discussed her daily eating habits in more detail. Although I am not a trained dietician or nutritionist, I think that most people understand the basic differences between eating a high-processed diet vs. a diet that consists of foods closest to their natural form (a.k.a. "whole foods"). I am not here to tell individual women what to eat. We all vary in our ability to tolerate various types of foods. But what you put in your mouth at each meal does influence your emotional and physical health. Most of the women who come to see me eventually notice a large container of Incredible Hulk-colored green liquid on my desk. I have even had new ladies come in telling me "Yes, I have heard from X, Y, or Z about your green drink." Now please don't jump to conclusions that I am some health-nut and that I run marathons in my free time. Nope, I'm simply a woman who, on working days, is too lazy to chew. What?! Yup, that's exactly right. On super busy days, I would rather drink my veggies; chewing a huge salad just takes too long.

I don't think that anyone, especially Popeye or your mother, can argue that we all shouldn't eat more veggies, especially greens. So why don't we do it? Because it takes time, can't typically be purchased at a drive-thru window, and often takes some motivation to figure out a new way to make string beans appealing. So how can we get around all of that? I finally decided to get one of those small high-speed blenders- in-a -cup contraptions, I have a NutriBullet, but there are many other brands available. In the morning, I just put in whatever I have in the fridge, add filtered water, and blend it all up. A typical morning will have a handful of spinach or kale, some parsley or cilantro springs, half a banana, half the juice of a lemon, a piece of ginger, water, and a healthy sprinkle of turmeric spice or actual turmeric root (for the anti-inflammatory properties).

For most people, this is an unflavored salad smashed through a blender, so it may not be at all palatable or remotely appealing. Do not worry. Luckily, I discovered Robyn Openshaw, www.greens-moothiegirl.com, who has a green smoothie recipe to satisfy most every palate. Julie was able to gain valuable guidance from Robyn's website about how to incorporate more whole foods into her and her family's daily meals. Julie was able to confidently say that just by slowly incorporating more "good" stuff into her diet, that she essentially naturally crowded out a lot of the processed, high-sugar, unhealthy "bad" stuff, and that her brain and body were responding positively. She started to understand what Robyn meant on her podcast "Your High Vibration Life" because in giving her body more of the vitamins, fiber, and micronutrients it needed, it started rewarding Julie with more energy, less fatigue, and more vitality. Julie could not have been more encouraged to continue what she had started because it finally resonated with her that she had not gone on some diet, but rather, had changed the way she nourished her body.

Sleep and Exercise

With her bathroom habits back on track with help from the probiotics and whole foods, we turned our attention to two more areas deserving of our attention in midlife: sleeping and exercising. Since Julie often reported waking up feeling unrefreshed most mornings, we decided to tackle that one first. While she could recall not having issues with sleep when she was in her 20s and 30s, she started feeling the effects of poor sleep in her early 40s. Again, there was no complaint of night sweats, which can often be problematic for women in the perimenopausal transition. Night sweats can lead to multiple wakings, often significantly disrupting sleep quality, which leads to daytime fatigue. She also denied symptoms of the major primary sleep disorders I typically screen for, such as obstructive sleep apnea and restless-leg syndrome.

Sleep

In exploring Julie's midlife sleep habits, it became clear that sleep had become a low priority, as she would often stay up late catching up on e-mails and Facebook into the wee hours of the morning. Prioritizing her sleep would be challenging but would yield positive results in many aspects of her life. So we decided to dig in and see what we could do to improve her current sleep debt.

As a society that values doing, we often dismiss rest as an unnecessary evil in a world that never slows down. We are lulled into thinking that we are somehow tougher, the less sleep we can get away with. That misconception is very harmful to our health and well-being, and we need to reconsider it.

Sleep is akin to plugging in our cell phones for recharging. We wouldn't dream of forgetting to charge our cell phones overnight so that they can perform for us the next day. Why don't we think of sleep as our human recharge? For our brains and bodies to heal and function optimally, we need this vital rest time to become a habit that we approach with loving attention and care. During sleep, our bodies go into a rest-and-repair state where various hormones and immune system functions go to work fixing whatever damage was acquired during the day. Various studies have demonstrated that chronic sleep deprivation can lead to weight gain by affecting blood sugar and insulin levels, causing cravings for sugary and fatty foods. Other studies show that lack of sleep affects brain health, leaving us feeling fatigued, foggy, or with impaired concentration. A better quality of life can be achieved when we make good sleep a priority.

I am often asked, "How many hours do I need to sleep?" No magic number fits every person. Some people feel they need 10 hours while others need 7. In general, sleep quality seems to be more important than sleep quantity. Even if you are technically in bed for 10 hours, but it is a poor-quality sleep, then you may feel just at good getting 7 to 8 hours if it is a deeper, more restorative sleep. So how do we go about improving the actual quality of our sleep? There are several strategies that I explore with patients, some of which may be more helpful to one person than another. If your goal is to improve your overall health and quality of life, it is worth trying all of these sleep techniques a few times to develop a personalized plan that works for you.

One of Julie's biggest issues was the evening time she spent on her electronic devices. She considered this her "special me-time" when there were no other distractions or demands from others, and she was not willing to give it up without a fight. Some things we discussed were related to blue-light exposure from her devices. I encouraged her to power them off at least an hour or two before she went to bed, but I realized that this would be challenging. Most cellular phones now have built-in blue-light filters that can be activated in the evening to limit blue-light exposure.

It is the blue light that tells our body that it is daytime, even when it's trying to secrete the sleep-inducing hormone melatonin to get us to sleep. We are confusing the heck out of our pineal gland (the tiny organ that produces melatonin in the brain) when we use our devices at a time our bodies want to be rejuvenating for the next day. In Julie's case, she used her computer to catch up on social media, so we discussed downloading F.LUX, a free program that alters your computer screen to encourage improved sleep rhythms. Even though these tips could be helpful, many people need to power off their electronic devices an hour or two before going to bed and engage in a calm activity like meditation, yoga, reading, or journaling. Some people say that can't fall asleep unless the television is playing in the background. But this, too, can lead to low sleep quality, and often causes multiple awakenings throughout the night leading to nonrestorative sleep.

The next thing we discussed was overall room darkness. I don't know about you, but even a night light or a street lamp shining a sliver of light into my bedroom disrupts my sleep. Julie admitted that her blinds, even when closed, did allow a considerable amount of light into her bedroom. While she did not want to invest in blackout drapes, she was willing to consider using a sleep mask that she put over her eyes when she went to bed. Most mornings, it was on the floor when she woke up, but she found that it did make it much easier to fall asleep. She liked this low-cost sleep tip and committed to using it nightly.

As Julie was already in the habit of brewing herself some night-time tea, we just discussed some formulations that have shown to help induce a relaxed state. She typically drank chamomile tea at night, but we also explored valerian and passionflower tea, both known for its relaxing effects. Julie also started taking a dose of magnesium nightly, which she felt relaxed her tense shoulder muscles. Magnesium is a muscle relaxer, which can help induce a more relaxed sleep and can be taken in a nightly dose of between 200 to 400 mg, according to www.peoplespharamacy.com. It is available in a pill form in all supermarkets and pharmacies, or in a powder form like in Thorne's Cal-Mag Citrate effervescent powder that you can mix in some water and drink.

Magnesium can be difficult to absorb, so some advocate taking it through the skin. Your skin is the largest organ in your body with a large surface area for absorption. You can take an evening bath in Epsom Salts or rub magnesium oil onto your skin before going to bed. Additionally, Julie started using an essential oil diffuser, alternating nights with either lavender or rose, which she felt calmed her as well. Even though she was not yet experiencing night sweats, she often felt that she was tossing and turning at night because her room felt hot and stifling. A cool room temperature can be helpful for a good night's sleep, so she invested in a portable fan than not only circulated the air but also provided her with needed cooling.

The final step in Julie's new and improved sleep plan was deciding on and sticking to a sleep schedule. We try to get kids on a consistent sleep schedule to allow them to rest and cut down on daytime crankiness. As adults, we also benefit from going to bed and getting up at the same time every day. Try it. This tip may help you get your sleep back on track.

Exercise

The final step in Julie's fatigue-fighting journey was related to moving and shaking her body on a regular basis. Now Julie was pretty vehement about the fact that she was not going to join a gym, nor was she going to start marathon training in her mid-40s. After talking about the options of what she could do, three things came to light. First, she had always dreamed of having one of those wide-seated cruiser bicycles but never thought she had the time to ride it or the money to buy it. Now she realized that instead of telling people to get her a gift card to a restaurant for Christmas or her birthday, that she could ask for help to buy a bike and helmet that she started to ride in a local park three times a week. She fell in love with the feeling of freedom cruising gave her, so she was inspired to make this a regular part of her body-love routine.

Second, she did own a pair of comfortable shoes and had a friend who has asked her if she wanted to walk sometimes, so she called her up and they walked once a week together to catch up. The final get-moving activity that Julie came up with was gardening. Her mother had been an avid gardener and had given her many of her gardening tools to Julie when she passed. Julie had just kept them boxed up in the garage, but in exploring the potential benefits of regular exercise on her fatigue, she found that she could also reconnect with a meaningful part of her family history.

In my time with Julie, although we were working on a specific goal to decrease her fatigue, all of the changes that she made gradually began to infuse her daily life with more energy and vitality. It was as if she had grown used to dragging through her day with little enjoyment and even less joy. This had become her status quo. Julie realized that she had embarked on a journey that had much more transformative potential than she had ever anticipated. The extra energy and motivation that she gained from these simple lifestyle changes allowed her to pursue a new hobby: training dogs to be service animals.

Additionally, she got more involved in the women's ministry at her church, an activity that allowed her to connect more deeply with a desire to be of service to others, but that she had avoided because of lack of life force as she entered midlife. Julie became renewed, inspired, and recharged, fully ready to tackle this stage of her gorgeous, newly inspired life. You go, girl!

CHAPTER 1 TIPS

1. Get your hormone levels checked.
2. Eat regularly to avoid hypoglycemia.
3. Consider gut health.
4. Add more whole foods to your diet.
5. Prioritize sleep.
6. Move your body.

CHAPTER 2

Who Am I and What Have You Done to My Brain?

I am not an early bird or a night owl. I am some form of permanently exhausted pigeon.

UNKNOWN

I can't quite tell you the exact moment my midlife body started telling me something was physically wrong. It was more like a gradual onset of brain fogginess, initially subtle, and remedied with a double espresso, which eventually progressed to four double espressos a day. I can recall a particular lunch date with a colleague who was enthusiastically telling me about the big plans she was developing to expand her business and all I could think was, "How does she have the energy for all that? What is wrong with me? I can barely make it through my day and am collapsing into bed by 8:00 pm!"

I was horrified when I heard myself utter the words, "And WHY would you want to do that?" I was shocked that in my brain fog, that was all the encouragement I could muster in response to her amazing news. I felt like a horrible friend. She looked at me and said, "Are you okay?" And I had to tell her no, that I was bone tired all the time, was gaining weight, and felt like my brain had cobwebs in it. Luckily, she looked at me with concern and said, "You need to check some labs. It sounds like your thyroid is out of whack."

Thyroid

Could my thyroid have taken a complete nosedive without me knowing it? That butterfly-shaped organ at the base of the neck affects virtually every cell in the body and controls many body functions. Its purpose is to make, store, and release thyroid hormones into the blood. My thyroid had decided to take a vacation and left my body up to its own devices without telling me.

A few days later, I was staring in disbelief at my abnormal lab values indicating that I was experiencing mild thyroid failure. I was exhibiting most of the adverse clinical consequences of low thyroid function, including fatigue, weakness, brain fog, coarse and dry straw-like hair, difficulty concentrating, weight gain, and cold intolerance. So, I was not a terrible, unsupportive friend after all? Thank goodness that I could blame this one on something that was happening to my body.

A couple of days after starting treatment, a tiny pill of replacement thyroid hormone, the brain fog started to lift. I eagerly texted my friend, asking her if this improvement could be just a placebo effect. "No," she said, "Some people feel better after a few doses of levothyroxine." All I could say was "Hallelujah" that my friend had called me out on my unsupportive comment and recognized that it was way out of character for me to behave like that.

Now for some statistics about thyroid dysfunction in midlife women.

1. In the Study of Women's Health Across the Nation, almost 1 in 10 midlife women had some abnormality of thyroid-stimulating hormone (TSH). Thyroid disease, one of the most common endocrine disorders in women, can be particularly challenging to diagnose when presenting at midlife (age range, 40 to 60)

because many symptoms of thyroid dysfunction can overlap with those of the menopausal transition, including menstrual changes, fatigue, sleep disturbances, changes in mood, skin and hair, and heat intolerance.

2. A family history of thyroid disorders, personal history of postpartum thyroiditis (an acute inflammatory state affecting some vulnerable women after delivery), previous treatment of Graves' disease (an autoimmune disorder of the thyroid), or other autoimmune disorders, such as type 1 diabetes, can increase the likelihood of developing thyroid dysfunction. How can women find out if their brain fog is associated with thyroid dysfunction?

3. Screening recommendations specific for women vary among expert groups, but all allow for increased suspicion and aggressive case finding in older women (especially those women with incidental findings on clinical interview or exam suggestive of thyroid disease.) For example, if you not only complain of brain fog, but you also have a head of coarse, dry, scarecrow hair, and you are sitting in the doctor's office in August in a down jacket because you are constantly freezing, you may be looking at a quick trip to the phlebotomist to get some lab tests drawn.

Auto-immunity

In my situation, I did not have a family history of thyroid dysfunction. I wondered if my problematic thyroid was trying to tell me, "your body is struggling." In looking at the staggering number of people in the U.S. and the world dealing with symptoms of auto-immunity, from Hashimoto's thyroiditis to Multiple Sclerosis, I started digging more deeply into this alarming phenomenon significantly affecting the quality of people's lives. I came across the work of Dr. Tom O'Bryan of the Betrayal Series and founder of TheDr.com. When he lost his father, he became motivated to find a more comprehensive way to evaluate physical symptoms and treat them from a functional medicine perspective. The Betrayal Series presented interviews with scientists, clinicians, and patients attempting to present a more whole-body approach to dealing with symptoms of autoimmunity. I started to look at the patients who would come to see me in a whole new light, a holistic, whole-body light, partly because of my health journey and partly because of what I learned from Dr. O'Bryan and his docuseries.

Thyroid Conditions/Hashimoto's Thyroiditis

Is it enough for your doctor to just order a TSH (thyroid-stimulating hormone) test to see what your thyroid may be doing? If you ask Dr. Isabella Wentz, www.thyroidpharmacist.com, you will hear a vehement "no." Dr. Wentz, a PhD pharmacist who, due to her struggles with hypothyroidism, has made it her life mission to educate people and health care practitioners about a more comprehensive way to evaluate a possibly underactive thyroid. It took her many years of debilitating symptoms to finally get to the cause of her symptoms, Hashimoto's thyroiditis, and many more years after her diagnosis to heal from her autoimmune condition. She believes that people need to ask their physicians to dig deeper than the common TSH test if they suspect that they are dealing with a thyroid problem. Why? Dr. Wentz believes that treatment for this type of underactive thyroid problem needs to be tackled from a cause perspective, not simply by giving a thyroid supplement in the form of thyroid hormone replacement, like synthetic levothyroxine or Armour thyroid, made from pig-derived thyroid glands.

At the minimum, in her website article, "Top 10 Thyroid Tests and How to Interpret Them," Dr. Wentz recommends that you ask your health care practitioner to order the following blood tests: TSH, Free T4, Free T3, TPO Antibodies, and TG Antibodies, to name the top 5. The reason for going beyond the traditional screening test of TSH is to make sure that an autoimmune cause for an underacting thyroid does not go unnoticed. On to her website, Dr. Wentz asks, "Did you know that 95% of those that are hypothyroid may have Hashimoto's?" As a physician and someone with hypothyroidism, I sheepishly admit that I didn't know this statistic. Now that I know, I look for it in all of the women whom I suspect may have low thyroid function.

Dr. Wentz believes that her root-cause approach for treating Hashimoto's thyroiditis, although involving many specific lifestyle modifications, like changing diet, dealing with stress, and taking thyroid-specific supplements, ultimately allows people to regain a quality of life and helps to prevent them for developing other autoimmune conditions. According to Dr. Wentz and other experts in the field of autoimmunity, once you have been diagnosed with one autoimmune disease, you are at greater risk of developing a subsequent one. Getting to the cause, not just treating the symptom, may allow you to lead a more healthful and vibrant life. Who doesn't want that?

Melinda's Story

When Melinda, a single woman in her mid-50s, came to see me, her chief complaint was "I'm anxious." In exploring her history, I learned that she had been a successful businesswoman, daughter, and super aunt to her niece for her entire life. Shortly after a trip to the East Coast, her family experienced a tragedy. It was so stressful that Melinda experienced her first panic attack. In addition to the ongoing family stress, she was experiencing physical symptoms like heart palpitations, dizziness, and feelings of uncertainty about her ability to cope with basic daily tasks, like grocery shopping or meal prep.

Anxiety

Before she was sent to me, the psychiatrist, she had undergone an exhaustive traditional medical work-up with visits to an internist, cardiologist, neurologist, and gastroenterologist, to name a few. Each physician had run tests, done lab work, and told her, "There is nothing wrong with you. You have anxiety. Go see a psychiatrist." So, she listened to what they said, and she came to see me.

I am often the last stop on an exhaustive health journey that women sometimes unexpectedly find themselves on. I often meet these women when they are frustrated, rejected, isolated, and made to feel like they are "crazy," to put it bluntly. It is the proverbial "Your symptoms are in your head. Go see the shrink" scenario. Ugh!

It always brings back an experience I had as a patient. I consulted a senior physician about a college-sport-related chronic back injury. At one point, he patted me on the back of my hand, saying, "Don't worry, honey. You should be able to bear children just fine." What? I was in there for an orthopedic consult, and someone was telling me about my childbearing potential? What did one thing have to do with the other? To this day, I am still not sure. I left that office and never went back. Many well-meaning practitioners dismiss women's symptoms, are condescending, or don't have the time or patience to dig deeper into their medical history, so they send these women to see a psychiatrist.

After discussing the trajectory of Melinda's symptoms, I couldn't ignore the nagging feeling that she was not experiencing classic anxiety symptoms. They felt more organic, like something medical caused them, rather than being "psychiatric." She tried numerous psychotropic medications traditionally used to treat anxiety, like SSRI (Selective-Serotonin Reuptake Inhibitors) or SNRI (Serotonin-Norepinephrine Reuptake Inhibitors). She experienced considerable side-effects and little to no relief from her "anxiety" symptoms.

In Melinda's situation, we decided to do genetic saliva testing to see how she metabolized medications, and the results showed that she likely poorly tolerate most serotonin-based medications, so it was not surprising that traditional pharmaceuticals for anxiety had provided little symptom relief. Additionally, we tested her for a genetic variation in the MTHFR gene, the gene responsible for converting inactive folic acid to the active form. Melinda tested negative for the MTHFR genetic variation, but I have had women who tested positive and benefitted from supplementing with a form of methylated folate.

The active form of folic acid is needed to produce the brain chemicals called neurotransmitters. Serotonin is an example of a neurotransmitter implicated in depression and anxiety. Sometimes people who have a single or double mutation in the MTHFR gene have more difficulty responding to medications for anxiety or depression and benefit from supplementation with l-methyl folate. It is the methylation that allows the folic acid to cross the blood-brain barrier serving as the building blocks for these natural brain chemicals. This MTHFR gene mutation is relatively common in the general population, and not many people know they have it. Because deficiency is so prevalent, practitioners will sometimes start someone on l-methyl folate supplementation without doing formal testing to see if symptoms improve in their depressed or anxious patients.

Identifying the Root Cause of Psychiatric Symptoms

In my work with Melinda, what became most apparent was that we were not likely to find the "perfect" medication to treat her anxiety symptoms because I did not think such a medication existed. She began the supplementation with l-methylfolate but was only able to tolerate very low doses, so it was unclear if she would get much benefit from the supplementation. Again, my intuition/gut was telling me that there was something else going on. I felt that something was going on with her immune system, similar to what had happened to me all those years ago. She was manifesting symptoms of her body trying to heal. I felt that our focus needed to be not on anti-anxiety medications, but on ways to support her immune system's ability to heal itself.

Through my healing journey, and in delving into the work of Dr. Terry Wahls, I knew that Melinda's body needed to be supported in a different way to heal than the traditional "take this pill and feel better" approach. Dr. Wahls was a physician who was diagnosed with secondary, progressive multiple sclerosis (an autoimmune disorder) and developed the Wahls' Protocol www.terrywahls.com. The Wahls' Protocol is a radical new way to treat all chronic autoimmune conditions using Paleo Principles and Functional Medicine.

Melinda's journey highlights a very important message to all women. As both a physician and patient, I know firsthand how it feels to have one's symptoms dismissed. This minimization can have two main outcomes. It can push someone to a place of isolation and despair where they accept what health care providers say as absolute truth. Or it can motivate someone to take radical action towards achieving health. For Melinda and me, during our initial health struggles, it was a bit of both initially. Ultimately, it started both of us on a journey of healing that would not have happened had we just accepted the status quo.

I want to encourage any woman reading this to not settle for leaving a doctor's office confused, conflicted, or dismissed. For me, the dismissal by a fellow physician triggered anger that boosted my resolve even more. I thought to myself that he might have given up on me, but I refused to give up on myself. For Melinda, it was a similar experience of recognizing that she was not ready to give up on a life that still had so much potential for happiness. She and I discussed all the things that she still wanted to do, and she was determined to do anything in her power to make those things happen.

One of the most critical aspects to explore and understand was the concept of time. Whatever was going on in Melinda's body had most likely been brewing for a while before she experienced her first physical symptoms. This is not the case in accidents or other emergent medical situations but can be the case for smoldering stealth attacks on our immune systems. We are living in a very different world now, where myriad environmental and chemical exposures, pesticides, and hormones in our food supply and increasing levels of stress undoubtedly are messing with our genes and our immunity, making us vulnerable to disease. Initially, it seemed overwhelming to revamp her entire lifestyle. But Melinda started chipping away at it bit by bit. We determined what the overriding theme was that Melinda wanted for this stage of her life. She said, "I want to be healthy and vibrant again." Once she stated that life goal, everything fell into place.

Nutrition as Medicine

We started with nutrition. The one thing that we all have direct control over is what we choose to put in our mouths each day. In Melinda's case, she underwent allergy testing to determine foods she might be sensitive to. In most cases, elaborate food sensitivity testing is not necessary. If people are willing to participate in a 4-week elimination protocol, they can see a pretty dramatic effect of nutrition on immune-system function.

Many physicians, nutritionists, and health care professionals are speaking to the power of revamping our nutritional status to improve physical and mental health. The biggest question I get asked is, "What is the best diet for me?" Most of us, undoubtedly, are confused about what to eat, given that there is a constant flood of articles, news stories, or books touting the latest and greatest superfood or way of eating. I do not believe there is a one-size-fits-all food plan. Just like everything else in life, determining the best foods for our bodies has to come from a gentle exploration of what foods work and don't work for each person.

The simplest way to ask your body for feedback is to get rid of some things for a few weeks and then slowly reintroduce them one at a time, listening to what your body is telling you. For example, for women coming in complaining of low energy, low vitality, and foggy brain, and are looking for an antidepressant, I will ask them first to consider putting aside gluten, dairy, and sugar for a month. What? I hear it all, "I can't give up milk. I crave it. What am I going to eat if I can't have bread and pasta? I am addicted to sugar and can't imagine not having my afternoon candy bar pick me up."

Often, this conversation must happen a few more times before someone is willing to see the potential of how differently their body and brain can feel just by tweaking some things. I am patient, and I don't give up. I imagine I sound like a broken record, but I know firsthand how revamping what I eat has done for my vitality, and I truly want women to experience this too.

How does one get started? For Melinda, it was just a day she picked to commit to the four-week no-gluten, dairy, and sugar life-style. She decided that four weeks out of her entire life was not that much to ask, especially if she could experience firsthand how her body could feel differently without these potential immune- system disruptors. With her overriding theme of health guiding her daily decisions, she would look at a food or a daily choice and say to herself, "Is eating or doing this in alignment with my goal of better health and vitality?" If the answer was no, she avoided it.

For example, when faced with the choice to sit down and watch mindless TV after work or put a leash on her dog and take a 20-minute walk around the block, she eventually began to recognize the choices that were health-promoting vs. health-sabotaging by choosing to focus on how engaging in certain activities made her feel. The equation became quite clear; sitting around made her feel bad and moving around made her feel better. It was a no-brainer, but as anyone knows, just because something is good for you, doesn't mean we will choose it.

Developing Healthier Habits

There are many articles written about how our brain chooses one option over another. We are pretty much wired to choose what is easier and expend the least amount of precious energy. So, don't be so hard on yourself if the couch feels like it is calling to you and the walk seems like torture after a long day at work. This stems from basic survival instincts, where choices that required more of us were considered riskier for our overall survival and were thus avoided. This means choosing to walk the dog instead of sitting and binge-watching the latest HBO series. We are required to tap into our higher cognitive centers. These are the same parts of our brains that we ask people to engage in the form of psychotherapy called CBT (Cognitive-Behavioral Therapy).

In CBT, you learn to challenge certain automatic thought patterns. For example, "I am never going to feel better, so why bother trying to exercise?" The CBT therapist would gently attempt to challenge that belief and help someone come up with other possible thought patterns to replace that one. For example, "If I never attempt to go for a walk, I will not know how it could make me feel." Homework is assigned, and the client is asked to engage in behaviors that challenge that original negative cognition. Eventually, one can experience a thought, challenge the validity of it, and employ an alternative ending.

The same thing would happen with food. When faced with the choice of having macaroni and cheese or roasted sweet potatoes, Melinda opted for the roasted vegetables because they were more in alignment with her life goal. Eventually, she was able to do the cognitive restructuring herself. She took a thought like, "I'm overweight already, so I should just eat whatever I feel helps relieve my stress" and converted it to "I may be overweight now, but if I choose a salad over a cheeseburger with fries enough times, I will lose weight and have more energy." What she noticed over time was that the good health choices began to crowd out the less healthy ones and that she began to notice positive changes in her energy, motivation, and vitality.

What made these subtle shifts stick was that she was doing it on her terms, at her own pace, treating herself with a kindness and gentleness that she had not done before. In the past, there had almost been a war with her body, punishing it by restricting what she ate, putting pills in it to lose weight, and drinking alcohol to numb memories of past sexual abuse. Now there was a sense of cooperation, forgiveness, and reverence for herself, her body, and her soul. There was an evolving sense that she and her body deserved to be loved and that this acceptance of her innate feminine fierceness would forever shift her sense of herself in her skin.

At 54, Melinda was reclaiming her body. The rest of her life was going to be the best of her life because she was living in alignment with a new vision for herself. Melinda became the powerful force of womanhood that she was meant to be because she decided to take back control over her daily life choices, instead of numbing herself with unhealthy food and defeating lifestyle practices and settling for a suboptimal existence.

Are you ready to align yourself with a new vision for your future? Whether you are trying to heal your underperforming thyroid like I was, or you are trying to boost your struggling immune system through a nutritional and detoxification approach like the Wahls' Protocol, the time is now to prioritize health, wellness, and vitality. You deserve this and much more, so please take a moment to consider the potential for reclaiming your life and your health by aligning yourself with body healing and supporting choices, rather than the usual default methods for coping with the stuff of life. Today is the first day of the rest of your life. Take at least one health-promoting step today and watch the good push out the bad, one choice at a time.

1   Since then, screening recommendations specific to women have varied by expert groups, but all allow for increased suspicion and aggressive case finding in older women (particularly those with incidental findings suggestive of thyroid disease). See more at: http://www.jwatch.org/na34807/2014/06/24/thyroid-disease-women-midlife#sthash.diuZj82r.dpuf

2   In the Study of Women's Health Across the Nation, almost 1 in 10 midlife women had some abnormality of thyroid-stimulating hormone (TSH). Family history of thyroid disorders, personal history of postpartum thyroiditis, previous treatment for Graves disease, or autoimmune disorders, such as type 1 diabetes, increase the likelihood of developing thyroid dysfunction. See more at: http://www.jwatch.org/na34807/2014/06/24/thyroid-disease-women-midlife#sthash.diuZj82r.dpuf

CHAPTER 2 TIPS

1. Ask your doctor to go beyond the TSH blood test when evaluating your thyroid.

2. Consider getting tested for the MTHFR genetic mutation if struggling with depressive or anxiety symptoms.

3. Try incorporating foods that help combat inflammation in the body.

4. Challenge negative thought patterns by being your own best therapist.

5. Be patient and treat your body with kindness and respect. It wants to heal, so try to help it do what it does best.

6. Each health-promoting step you take crowds out vitality-destroying habits.

The Looking Glass:
Your Body IS a Wonderland[1]

Not one drop of my self-worth depends on your acceptance of me.

QUINCY JONES

A h, the looking glass, otherwise referred to as the bathroom or compact mirror. I sometimes muse about a world without these shiny, reflective devices that come in every shape and size and seem to be just about everywhere one looks. Why does an elevator need to have floor-to-ceiling mirrors? The psychiatrist in me would suppose it might have something to do with preventing a claustrophobic panic attack. But the feminine instinct supports a more sinister plot: constantly checking ourselves out and comparing ourselves to our elevator neighbor. I seriously wonder if cavewomen cared about stubborn chin hairs needing plucking or if they were concerned that grey hairs were making their complexion appear washed out? I doubt it. Escaping from a woolly mammoth was probably a more pressing issue at the time. How times have changed.

---

1   John Mayer, singer-songwriter. "Your Body is a Wonderland." Oct. 2002.

Appearance

Fast forward to 2016, where Statista, the web-based statistics portal, cites annual revenue of the cosmetics industry to top $62.46 billion U.S. dollars this year alone. Now don't get me wrong. I, too, have a medicine cabinet, an under the sink cabinet, and a dedicated bathtub basket stuffed with various beauty creams and potions. I am a realist. I want to feel decent about myself, my hygiene, and not be mistaken for a crocodile come winter. However, with the passage of time, I realize that keeping up with the Kardashians might be easier than keeping up with the onslaught of recommendations for "staying youthful" or "turning back time." It would be a full-time job to keep up with the latest and greatest advancements in anti-aging, and I'm not convinced that is the best use of my waking portions of the average 24-hour day. Honestly, I would rather take a nap.

In my work with women, I know that each of us has a unique comfort level with what we are willing to present to the outside world. I, too, will make an effort to pull myself together in a different way when going to work versus a Sunday afternoon spent in sweat-pants. This is normal. Some of us will still do full hair and makeup, even on sweatpants Sunday, and that is okay too. I think it is more important for us to respect each other and not judge what we each to do to feel good in our skin. We have all our unique history, and we do what makes us feel most confident to function optimally in our daily lives.

There are situations, however, where the desire to look younger has gone awry. In the condition known as Body Dysmorphic Disorder or BDD, a mental illness that the latest edition of the DSM-V (the *Diagnostic and Statistical Manual, 5th edition*) classifies as a type of obsessive-compulsive disorder (OCD). BDD sufferers experience extreme levels of anxiety over real or imagined physical flaws. This mental health condition is very different from our typical occasional female insecurities about our appearance. People suffering from BDD are obsessed and chronically anxious about their perceived defect or defects to the point that their quality of life and daily functioning is significantly impaired. They may lead to repetitive behaviors, such as excessive grooming rituals and repeated cosmetic surgeries that can become so time-consuming, that it often becomes impossible to maintain a job or social life. This is a relatively rare condition, occurring in about 2% of the U.S. population, but one in which it is very difficult to break free without professional support and help.

So, what really what happens when a midlife woman looks into her daily looking glass? As we have just seen, the range of experiences can vary from nonchalance to a weekly standing appointment with one's cosmetic dermatologist, hairdresser, manicurist, and personal trainer. Most of us probably fall somewhere in the middle. I have learned that I am quite impatient when it comes to grooming, so I have picked up many handy time-saving tricks of the trade to use in a pinch. Can you say $5 bottle of "hair-root rescue" or those handy $7 bottles of gel nail polish that don't look half bad two weeks after my home Pedi? We all have our habits, rituals, and feel-good tactics that work for us and I think that is the take-home message. We each need to do what works for us because wasting time comparing how we look at midlife in relation to another woman is just plain silly.

Why, for example, are we always curious to find how old another woman is? I admit that I was one of those people too, although I started trying to understand what makes me want to do that. As human beings, there is a natural tendency to look towards others and do some self-comparisons. If that motivates you to do better in some area of your life, then that is great. For example, if I see a woman doing something inspirational, like running her first marathon after beating breast cancer, that makes me push myself to at least take that 15-minute walk on the treadmill, even if I am bone tired and would rather sit and read a magazine. Looking at each other with admiration and compassion at any life stage will always serve us much better as a community of women than judging and being critical of where each of us is on our life journey. I'm not saying we shouldn't put on some blush and mascara tomorrow if we want to, but we can work on being more mindful about approaching our fellow midlifers with a more open and accepting heart. This will only come if we first work on being more loving and compassionate with ourselves.

Mindfulness

How do we do that? How do we become able to greet these changes in the looking glass without having a significant and profound mood dip? I can't speak for everyone, but for me, daily meditation practice has helped. No, I am not asking you to move to Tibet or even to spend hours a day in a pretzel pose, repeating a mantra over and over under your breath. I am just talking about cultivating a wider perspective on daily life. Many incredible teachers have devoted their lives to encouraging others to live more mindfully, and we have all come across their famous quotes here and there throughout life. But it was not until I embarked on a personal and professional quest to learn more about the transformative potential of this way of life, that I had my "a-ha" moment about how this could help me and my patients navigate the stuff of midlife and beyond.

There are countless incredible people like His Holiness, the Dali Lama and Thich Nhat Hahn, the Vietnamese Buddhist monk who coined the term "Engaged Buddhism," who have offered a modern light on meditation practice. Dr. Kristin Neff, a pioneering self-compassion researcher, and Dr. Jon Kabat-Zinn, creator of the Stress Reduction Clinic and the Center for Mindfulness in Medicine, are both leaders in the field of applying strategies of more conscious, in-the-present-moment based living. This is allowing people to break free from old patterns by embracing novel methods of thinking about themselves and the world. It helps us better cope with stress, anxiety, pain, and illness. With a nod towards the simple and practical, these teachers bring our attention from society's hyper-driven focus on the exterior, towards what matters on the interior.

I know that moving away from an emphasis on the looking glass as we enter this period of our lives will certainly benefit us by bolstering our resiliency in the coming years. Plus, it will save you a lot of money in the long run. Think of all the $300 caviar face creams and Botox injections you'll be able to pass on now that you have given daily mindfulness practice a front row seat in your life. You can thank me later.

Michelle's Story

Michelle, a 42-year-old African-American breast cancer survivor, was referred by her internist after she admitted to her doctor that she was having trouble adjusting to life after her active cancer treatment had ended. People who have not personally been touched by cancer, or have a loved one who has been through this, may misunderstand the concept of survivorship. The most common response is, "Well, your treatment is over, isn't that great?" or "It's all behind you now, so why aren't you happy?" Active treatment is just one part of the overall cancer journey. Many people are cured of their cancer by treatment modalities like chemotherapy, radiation, and stem-cell transplants, but that is often just the tip of the iceberg. Living with the side effects of the various treatments and trying to piece back a life that is not consumed by disability, dysfunction, or grief is not for the faint of heart.

Body Changes

For Michelle, the challenges of adjusting to a body radically changed by her breast cancer treatment were daunting. She was still experiencing pain where she had lymph nodes removed, and she was forced to wear an arm sleeve to contain the lymphedema (chronic swelling related to reaccumulating lymphatic fluid after surgical lymph node removal). She was battling hot flashes from the Tamoxifen she was taking, and she was feeling dissatisfied with her weight gain as a result of fatigue and food choices she had been making over the stressful and hectic course of cancer treatment. All these bodily changes were wreaking havoc on her self-esteem. They challenged everything she knew about herself from her intimate relationship with her partner to her friendships. Some had been supportive, and others had been less so. She was hoping that being declared cancer free by her oncologist would have afforded her a sense of lightness of being she had not experienced for the year of her active cancer treatment. Instead, she found herself on yet another uphill battle of mourning her sense of being betrayed by her body and needing to make it her friend again, not an enemy to loathe and hold at a distance.

Her body's betrayal became the initial focus of our discussions. Most people would describe Michelle's lifestyle as healthy: no smoking, a glass of wine socially once a month, a jog around the park three times a week, a diet filled with many salads, and at least 7 to 8 hours of sleep nightly. It took her many hours of educating herself during her long hours receiving chemotherapy that breast cancer can strike, even if you are doing everything "right."

To some degree, she had worked through much of that before she came to me. What was challenging her about her body now was the unexpected changes that treatment had produced, namely the lymphedema and weight gain. She admitted that she could not even look at herself in the mirror anymore and avoided looking down at her body when bathing or showering. It was just too painful and made her tear up and cry when she focused on what her body had become.

We had to sit for a long while with the deep, heavy feelings of grief over a body that was forever changed through this battle with breast cancer before we could hope to move towards any possibility of forgiveness or healing. She talked to her body in session with me, would journal to her body at home, and even painted her body in the various ways she remembered it from the past and how it was today.

When she felt ready, she began to slowly melt the fear of connecting with her brokenness by just hugging herself and thanking her body for withstanding the intense treatment protocol and allowing her to be alive for her family today. Eventually, she would stand in front of the bathroom mirror and kindly, tenderly, lovingly touch her heart, arm, reconstructed breast, and whisper, "thank you, body, for not giving up on me. I love you." This journey of reclaiming her sense of love for the body that had enjoyed sexual intimacy with her partner, completed two half-marathons, and survived breast cancer was slow, difficult, and lonely. The truth, though, was that she was far from being alone.

Just like with many things that women go through across the lifecycle, talking about cancer survivorship as relates to our sexual selves is not discussed with most oncologists, who understandably are focused on the cure, rather than on helping pick up the pieces left by treatment. Some medical doctors are aware of the physical and emotional implications of the various treatment modalities currently being employed in Western approaches towards cancer treatment. But there are time limitations, increasing patient loads, and the management of very sick patients that often preclude this conversation about how to thrive as a woman in survivorship. It is time that we, as women begin, to demand these discussions with our health care providers, as integrating the sum of our parts into a whole-body approach is the only road to true wholeness, body, and mind. Are we ready to start a revolution? I know I am. How about you?

Perspective Shifts

Much of the work that I do with women around our changing bodies is related to perspective shifts. What exactly does that mean? Well, in simplest terms, it is kind of like that proverbial question, "Is this glass half full or half empty?" I try to meet a woman where she is with the response to that simple question and bring it up a notch. If she says the glass is half full, then I can take a quiet sigh of relief, knowing that helping her with perspective shifting may be a bit easier. However, if she is viewing the same glass as half empty, I have my work cut out for me. Yes, you can argue that I am overgeneralizing quite a bit with this example. However, you would be surprised at how telling the response is in the grand scheme of a woman's vision of herself and her life.

Another way I often describe it to patients is by using the analogy of a car filter. When your mechanic inserts a shiny, new, spotless filter into your car, it works great. The car runs smoothly, and everything flows and works effortlessly. As time goes on, however, dirt, grime, and pollutants start to contaminate and alter the filter, so that it is still functioning, but sub-optimally. Eventually, if we do not go back for a sparkly new car filter, our car will struggle to work properly and eventually give out on us when we need it to get us somewhere.

Our brain and body filters work the same way. When we are born, for the most part, we have a pretty clean slate. Depending on our childhood and other life experiences, our filter can remain relatively clear, or with each situation of abuse, hardship, illness, loss, or betrayal, can get muddy, darker, and more difficult to see through. Eventually, even our current life experiences begin to be filtered through this damaged, worn filter, often undermining our potential to experience the fullness of life's joy. My job is to understand a woman's history—her filter—and see what cleaning needs to happen so that she may begin to see things differently.

At the end of each new evaluation, I take a moment to acknowledge the courage that it must have took to come in to see me. For some women, scheduling an appointment with a psychiatrist may not be more stressful than getting their nails done, and that is great. For everyone else, including me, I would have to be feeling pretty darn bad to be vulnerable enough to see a perfect stranger and spill my guts. Empathy and our shared humanity force me to acknowledge that whatever drove her to come in to see me—whether it be courage, curiosity, or desperation—each is equally impressive and needs to be verbalized and understood. True transformation and healing are most likely when we share another person's deepest vulnerabilities and fears. My goal is to have women be cleansed of all that is holding them back from the full life they deserve. It is a sacred relationship that I am humbled to partake in.

CHAPTER 3 TIPS

1. Just do you. Comparing yourself to other women leaves you feeling half empty.

2. Celebrate being alive every day. An attitude of gratitude always trumps negativity.

3. Cultivate loving-kindness towards yourself first and when you master that, then towards others.

4. Thank your body for being there for you in the here and now, and forgive it when it is hurting, or you feel it has disappointed you.

5. If you don't feel understood by your treatment provider, don't be afraid to go elsewhere to meet your care needs.

6. We are all in this together. Spread a little empathy everywhere you go, and you'll be surprised at how connected you to feel to the sisterhood around you.

CHAPTER 4

Gerber Baby to Graduate

Raising children is a creative endeavor, an art rather than a science.

BRUNO BETTELHEIM

With the advancement of fertility treatments, many more women have been having their first Gerber moment in midlife. They are joining women on crowded playgrounds who either started their journey into motherhood earlier, adopted, blended families, or who, in the process of expanding their brood, are spacing out children. Let's not forget the friends having a "surprise" 40th Birthday present arrive nine months after their celebratory getaway weekend. Anyway, you have created a family in your life, juggling the needs of your kiddos with the changing needs of your midlife body and brain can sometimes be tricky. Remember that you are not alone, especially when you start to get those overwhelming feelings that are normal for modern-day motherhood.

How can we be expected to keep track of the latest and greatest in baby gear while still remembering to show up at school for our middle-school child, who is exhibiting her erupting volcano in the Science Fair? I remember spending the entire day roaming through the acres of fields and farmland around our home in Pennsylvania growing up. My parents said, "See you around dinner time," and off

I went. I did not have an iPhone or a Blackberry to text them, nor did they have a GPS unit tracking my exact location. I was a kid growing up in suburbia in the late 70s/early 80s, and my parents had no reason to fear the worst each time I went through the front door.

Helicopter Parenting

Fast forward to the present, where the culture of anxiety, danger, and worst-case scenarios permeates the modern parent's existence and dampens the modern's child sense of self-efficacy. I am as guilty of this mindset as the next person who responsible for the safety and wellbeing of a child. I admit that I do not let my kids out the door with a cheery, "See you at dinnertime, kids!" It's more like, "Okay, go out and play in the backyard and I'll watch you with one eye as I wash the dishes." Is this irrational behavior on my part going to change anytime soon? Probably not. But we need to strike a healthier balance between tempering our need to somehow control the outcome of everything (impossible, as you may already know) and allowing kids to learn to be more confident and resilient. Yes, bad things sometimes happen and that is devastating, but I know that the few times my younger son injured himself to the point of passing out in pain was right in front of me.

I can recount every last detail of the four times that I was shaking him awake saying, "Are you okay?" He was. These things do not happen as often now. Is it because he is older and wiser at 14 years and he is making better choices? Or is it because I am taking bigger emotional leaps of faith and am letting him be a kid like I was all those years ago? I don't know exactly, but I know that as I age, I am slowly letting go of the idea that I am somehow in control of this thing called life.

For all of you who have an infant, toddler, or young child in your life, I am preaching to the choir. It is your job to be overly cautious to the point of being a little OCD for about those first 10 or so years.

What is probably more important than being extra careful about their safety and care is not forgetting to nurture yourself along the way. "What?!" I can almost hear you exclaim; "I don't have time for myself, let alone time for all of the things that I have to do today." Yes, I completely understand, but I also spend much of my time helping women try to dig themselves out of mood and anxiety states that have taken over their brains and lives.

Genetics

We know that some of these conditions may be partly related to our genetics. Many studies indicate that what we inherit from our families is one factor that increases our vulnerability to brain strain, and emotional and mental illness. I am not minimizing the role of genetics in any way. I want to highlight that while the genetic lottery is largely out of our control, we can try to have more of a say as to the other variables that affect emotional well-being.

There is a lot of interest in the phenomenon of epigenetics, as it related to the expression of certain genes we may inherit. As we go through life, we are exposed to environmental situations that can trigger hormonal changes that can either activate or silence certain genes. According to an article by Kanherkar et al., "Epigenetics Across the Human Lifespan," there is a constant interaction between our internal and external environments that influence disease load and resistance to illness. Exposure to various chemicals, toxins, stress, as well as diet, exercise, and other environmental factors, can bring about positive or negative epigenetic modifications that affect development, metabolism, and health.

In a nutshell, this means that regardless of what a family member may have suffered from during their lifetime, we can influence the expression of genes that may have been activated in our loved one and keep them quiet. I feel that this research can empower us to not succumb to beliefs such as, "Well, Mom/Grandmother had this, so I'm probably going to get it" mentality. That belief can be tremendously disempowering and harmful. If there is a way to affect a different and unexpected outcome in our lives by making some simple lifestyle changes, then why shouldn't we try?

The worst-case scenario would be that we get the disease or condition we've been dreading all along. Then again, the flip side may also be equally possible. By cleaning up our diets, starting to move our bodies daily in some way, engaging in a mindfulness practice to better manage stress, or making regular dates with a friend to decrease social isolation, we may be able to keep those disease genes from turning on. Along that journey of silencing bad genes through our lifestyle choices, we may end up enjoying many years with a higher quality of life, more contentment, and greater joy. What is stopping you from making even one change in your daily routine that has the potential to yield powerful positive outcomes?

Self-care in Motherhood

With our understanding that our daily choices affect our genes, motherhood is just one time in a woman's life that we should be paying closer attention to maintaining physical and emotional equi-librium. However, it seems that it is easier to focus on the self before kids and after they leave home. That time in between these two events is like the Bermuda Triangle of health. That mysterious space where lines blur between self and other. Of course, no one argues that this is an exceptional time in the lives of women, demanding physical and mental sacrifices akin to preparing oneself to a mission to the moon.

The main difference is that the average astronaut takes one of these missions in his or her lifetime. In contrast, the average woman caring for children is exposed to mental and physical wear and tear on a daily basis for many, many years. If she does not consider the potential for mission failure, if she does not minister to her physical and emotional needs on a daily basis, there may be a major physical or emotional meltdown at some point in the future.

Many of you may be asking yourselves, "What is she talking about? I'm doing just fine." Yes, I admit that, based on my career choice of psychiatry, I am slightly biased in my perspective. I am also a realist, and as a mother myself, I know that there is no one out there who has not had an off day at some point. However, if you are so genetically and environmentally blessed that there is nothing in your life that needs attention, then you can skip this chapter and maybe the rest of this book. I am truly and honestly happy for you. If you are like the rest of us, though, doing the best we can every day to face the challenges ahead with grace and stamina, then please read on.

Most of us, if not all, have had a day where between the juggling act of daily responsibilities, we may have wanted just to wave a white flag in surrender. This is otherwise known as, "I want to get an out of jail ticket for this thing called adulthood just for today, please." This is normal. You are okay.

Most of us think that having Wonder Woman days, where we effortlessly deflect daily stresses with our golden wristbands, is the norm or ideal to aspire to. I beg to differ. I cannot imagine how many hours sweet Linda Carter spent in hair, makeup, and wardrobe for every episode of her hit television series. I can tell you that the closest I come to that Wonder Woman image is the one time every couple of months I make an appointment with my hairdresser for a trim and blow out. Most of us are hopefully trying to strike a happy medium between looking like Wonder Woman and being a contestant roughing it on an episode of *Survivor*, each choosing to pay some degree of attention to our appearance as an integral part of a self-care routine.

One might argue "Why should one bother with pampering the exterior when the focus should be on our interior?" I am not here to argue what any woman should be doing or not doing with her physical appearance, given all of the cultural and societal pressures put on women. All of us should be free to choose how we want to express our individuality and femininity. Unfortunately, there is a lot more mind expansion that needs to happen on a global level to truly afford women many basic rights of self-expression.

I am mainly guided by the clinical interaction with the women who seek help on their journeys towards emotional wellness. My role is to meet each woman where she is at this moment, considering the unique aspects of her life story, and begin the gentle exploration of what needs to shift in her life to bring things into better balance. For the new mom battling postpartum depression, who has not been able to muster the precious energy required to shower and change out of the baby food stained sweatpants she has been wearing for three days straight, a greater focus on the physical aspects of self-care may be where we need to make a temporary pit stop. Ultimately, my job is to help a woman figure out the necessary choices she needs to make to propel herself towards wellness, in body and mind.

Carla's Story

Carla was a 46-year-old mother of two, a 17-year-old son and a 12-year-old daughter, who was referred to me by her OB/GYN because of symptoms of depression. She had tried several antidepressants over the years prescribed by various health care providers for complaints of depressed/low mood, irritability and anger, and low motivation. She had never seen a therapist or psychiatrist before. There was no family history of depression and reported medical issues.

Depression

When we started talking, it was quite obvious that Carla was struggling with symptoms of depression, but she was still functioning fairly well in her day-to-day life. She was able to attend to her daily tasks as a stay-at-home mom without much difficulty. She reported that her husband Tom provided well for the family and that her children were doing well in school. As we pieced together her history, I had this nagging feeling that she was not telling me something.

Carla presented neatly groomed and wearing a fashionable outfit, but there was something in her eyes that that was far more revealing than anything she could have told me. There was a detached, almost listless look to her gaze that would be evident whenever we touched upon an aspect of her family life.

Domestic Abuse

A standard question I ask is about any history of abuse: physical, sexual, emotional, or verbal. It wasn't until I said the words emotional and verbal that I noticed Carla inhale softly, yet sharply enough that it seemed unnatural. Initially, she responded "no" to all of the abuse questions, but something about her body language told me otherwise. She shifted in her seat and briefly looked away and down before her eyes settled back on mine.

I felt, in that moment of vulnerable intimacy, that I had to question her about this aspect of her history gently. I said, "I appreciate how difficult it is to come in and have to answer all of these personal questions. It would be hard for me to do so with someone I barely met, but we are going to be working together as a team moving forward, so I need us to be as honest as possible with each other, even if there is something scary or painful going on in your life. It is okay. I am here for you no matter what it is."

Carla's eyes welled up with tears, and her lips started to tremble. Her eyes were cast downwards, and she quietly whispered, "He yells at me. Calls me stupid. Checks my phone." She continued to stare at the ground, tears just streaming down her face. I reached across the desk, placed my hand on top of hers, and just held it there for a few moments. Then I said, "I am so sorry for what you are going through. You do not deserve what is happening to you. As hard as it was to tell me this, you owe it to you to speak the truth of what you are going through."

The statistics on domestic violence in the United States are staggering. According to the National Coalition Against Domestic Violence, on average, nearly 20 people per minute are physically abused by an intimate partner. One in three women have been victims of some form of physical violence by a partner in their life-time. In Carla's case, her husband had not been physically violent towards her, but had engaged in repeated episodes of verbal, emotional, and financial abuse.

When she and her husband met, Carla was working as an occupational therapist at a local health center. Within three months of getting married, Carla became pregnant with her first child, a daughter who was now 17 and getting ready to graduate from high school. Although she had enjoyed her job, she also looked forward to being a mom, and when she and her husband decided that she would stay home, she didn't think much of it because she was very excited at the prospect of new motherhood.

The first few years as a stay-at-home mom were extremely busy, and Carla's husband worked long hours as he made his way up the ranks as a pharmaceutical representative. When their second child was born, and her husband temporarily got laid off, financial strain began to cause strife in the household as Tom began to monitor Carla's spending, giving her a weekly allowance for groceries and other expenses that she was required to adhere to.

She was required weekly to provide him with her checkbook balance, and if she had not adhered to the allocated budget, Tom would get angry, call her dumb, and withhold money from her the following week as a form of punishment. Tom expected Carla to look well-groomed and well-dressed but required that she do so on his restricted budget. When she had difficulty losing weight after her second baby, Tom would criticize her weight, comparing her to other women he worked with and told her what to eat. When she was not successful, he would intentionally withdraw affection from her, telling her he would not be attracted to her unless she lost weight.

Even after things improved financially for the family with Tom's promotion, many of the dynamics between Tom and Carla were firmly entrenched. She tried to lose herself in raising the children, but as the time of her daughter leaving home grew near, Carla's sense of despair increased, thus fueling her reporting of depressive symptoms. In exploring Carla's history, she admitted that her mother, who had worked as a librarian and raised Carla and her two brothers, had also stopped working soon after her firstborn.

Carla recalled that her father, the sole breadwinner, had been critical of her mother, her appearance and cooking, and would limit her ability to have friendships. Things shifted dramatically when Carla's father suffered a stroke in his mid-50s and was forced to retire. At that point, Carla's mother went back to work. Even though Carla was about 12 when this happened, she noticed a change in how her mother and father interacted. Her mother took great pride in getting dressed up, driving the car to work, being appreciated and acknowledged for her hard work, and supporting the family financially. Her parents stayed married, and her mother worked until her early 70s when she finally decided to retire. As an adult, Carla noticed that her mother had become the head of the household, replacing her father who, due to his medical issues, had retreated into his world of isolation and depression.

Carla looked up, having been caught up in retelling this child-hood story and softly muttered "I never want to be treated like this again. I do not want to be financially dependent on anyone. I feel trapped, depressed, and broken. I need help." It was really at that moment of honesty with herself and her situation. The act of verbalizing it and putting it out into the universe caused something shifted inside of Carla. Her situation was veiled in so much secrecy that as she continued to carry the weight of this burden. It continued to fuel and magnify her symptoms of depression.

She would have continued trying new pills, attempting to medicate feelings that were the product of a dynamic that, up until this point, had seemed hopeless to change. Although Carla's situation was unique to her, this cycle of relationship challenges around motherhood and beyond is all too common. The struggles of some women who decide to embrace a new life path of stay-at-home motherhood wholeheartedly are real but rarely discussed. In many cases, the conflicts between a stay-at-home partner and one working outside of the home initially are subtle and often dismissed. Over time, these chronic frustrations erode a woman's sense of self.

Sense of Self During Motherhood

Having seen this too many times in my work, I have made a conscious effort to bring up the topic of a women's identity before and after children in the pregnant and postpartum moms I see. The main point in having these discussions is to allow women to understand that at any point in life, they are a sum of myriad intricate parts, many of which were put in place before they ventured into motherhood. Women can gently nurture these parts of themselves throughout motherhood, or these parts can be abandoned or buried. Abandoning parts of themselves can lead to a sense of identity confusion when their children become more independent and start flying the coop. Despite all the wishing to the contrary, they do leave.

I am already experiencing pieces of that realization as my sons become teenagers and grow excited about building their futures. We must have a little something that we call our very own slowly simmering on the backburner even while we invest deeply and lovingly in childrearing. The more we honor our whole self, the richer our ability to mother can be.

I already hear the complaints of "What? I don't have time to shower, so how am I going to do anything for myself? There are not enough hours in the day between laundry and carpool." I can relate. When my sons were first born, I decided to stay at home with them. I took an almost three-year sabbatical from work to take care of them. Yes, I was very fortunate to have a partner who was working and able to provide for us those years, and many women do not have that option. However, in between diaper changes, throwing something into the Crock-Pot, and forcing myself out of sweatpants, I would take a few minutes out of every day, usually when the kids were napping, and the laundry was spinning, to catch up on articles on the Internet about women's mental-health issues. I know, very exciting, huh? Yes, I am a nerd, I admit it. I digress.

The point is that especially during the times that I felt like I was drowning under the relentless stream of mommy responsibilities, I had enough will to keep myself afloat by doing at least a short daily check-in with the person I knew I had been (and still was) under the spit up that I was wearing. This anchor to my former self is what allowed me to embrace each long, adult-less day without losing it until my husband came through the door in the evening and I could hand off the kids to him for a bit.

This connection to something that was my very own—my love of psychiatry was a critical part of my growth as a woman, human, and mother. I always encourage women in my practice not to neglect important parts of themselves, no matter where they are on their life journey because we all deserve to feel self-love, personal satisfaction, and a deep sense of contentment with ourselves, no matter what we are facing in our day-to-day lives. For some patients, it has been nurturing a 15-minute daily yoga or meditation practice in between baby naps, keeping up their continuing education credits or licensing requirements, starting up an idea for a book, taking time to work on a painting, or exploring their love of cooking. No matter what ignites your innermost passions, keeping that flame alive will enable you to feel more grounded, contented, and whole, no matter how many piles of dirty laundry are staring you down.

In Carla's situation, she ended up forging a path similar to her mother's. After a handful of couple sessions, Carla and Tom agreed that she would start working at a local bakery on the weekends. Although she had enjoyed her work as an occupational therapist, she had always loved baking and wanted to explore that interest and still contribute financially to the household. With her daughter heading to college, they could use the extra income and her husband could take their son to his weekend baseball practices.

After about three months, Carla returned for a visit with a rejuvenated sense of self. She was smiling, not voicing depressive symptoms, and was so enjoying her part-time job (except for the 5 am wake-up call to bake the donuts) that she enrolled in an online culinary school's program to earn a baking certification. As Carla's confidence in her baking abilities grew, so did her resolve to start working on other aspects of herself that she had been neglecting: her health, friendships, and marriage.

She and Tom celebrated their 18th wedding anniversary with a gorgeous layer cake that she had created herself. I often remind the women I work with that we are all connected in our humanity, no matter what we are experiencing individually as women. When I said this to Carla, she reflected upon this and said, "I am so grateful that I took a chance on myself and came in to see you that day. It was like my OB/GYN had unknowingly thrown me a life ring when I was drowning by sending me to you. I got another chance at my life because you believed in me when I didn't believe in myself. Please share what I have gone through to encourage other women. They are worth it. Please let them know." Although Carla's journey was not always easy, the foundation that she rebuilt for herself was solid enough to carry her forward in her life, no matter what would lay ahead.

CHAPTER 4 TIPS

1. Control is an illusion. Anxiety robs you of your precious life force. Seek ways to trust more and worry less.

2. Our genes do not limit us. Take pro-active steps to be the pioneer of a new-and-improved family history.

3. Motherhood requires you to remember to put your oxygen mask on first before assisting others.

4. It's okay to want to spend a day under the covers. This is called self-care, and each one of us needs this once in a while.

5. If your partner is emotionally, verbally, or physically abusing you, know that you are not alone. Seek support. Each one of us needs to know our value and deserves to be respected.

6. Strive to connect regularly with something that ignites your passion or is meaningful to you. An unattended fire tends to burn out. Take the time to properly fuel the flame to provide a steady source of light and warmth in your soul.

CHAPTER 5

Family: To Each One's Own

I believe that the greatest gift you can give your family and the world is a healthy you.

JOYCE MEYERS

Each one of us was born to a mother. The rest of the story is as varied as there are stars in the sky. Whether we were adopted, orphaned, blended, or simply born and remained in our family of origin, our concept of what makes a family is our own. Each woman attempts to weave her unique history of the family into her concrete reality. Along the way, the imagined future usually undergoes several permutations. Some changes are welcomed, like when a toxic relationship dissolves for the best. Some changes are unwelcome, like when hopes for a healthy delivery go awry. In each of these situations, the capacity of women to cope, survive, and thrive is remarkable. It's the very reason why I devote my work to holding, processing, and moving through pain with the brave warrior women who seek collaboration with me.

Amy's Story

Amy, a 41-year-old mother, had been seeing me for help with generalized anxiety symptoms. Amy struggled with infertility for many years and had ultimately adopted a toddler, Sam. During our work together, she called excitedly one day with the news that she was pregnant. This joy, however, was short-lived. At the 8-week ultrasound, there was no heartbeat detected. Amy presented to me several weeks after this pregnancy loss, distressed and distraught. There was a frenzied look of pain, longing, and sorrow on her face. Her eyes were rimmed with red, swollen lids. She hollowly repeated the words, "It just doesn't seem real. One moment she was here, and now she is gone."

Pregnancy Loss

Amy already knew she had lost a beloved baby girl, having undergone blood testing that had revealed her baby's sex. There had not been enough time to process this loss. The emphasis was on making sure the fetus was removed from the uterus during a dilatation and curettage (D & C) procedure. She needed to handle the rest of the grief journey on her own.

We sat together as she quietly sobbed, shoulders hunched forward, tears flowing from her eyes like a sudden summer downpour. I felt, at that moment, a need to help her somehow get a firmer grasp on the reality of what had just happened. I excused myself and walked over to the ultrasound tech in our office and asked her to pull up and print out the last recorded image of Amy's baby. I brought this little black and white picture back into the room, sat next to her, and gave her the image. Amy sat, holding the photograph in both hands and looked up at me. She said, "This picture helps makes it feel real. I am NOT crazy. I am now sure that I carried her inside of me because for a moment, I thought I had imagined the whole thing."

This simple act turned out to be the pivotal piece of Amy's grief journey. She later explained that she put the picture in a frame and that having that as a concrete remembrance of her daughter's ever-so-fleeting existence helped anchor this child in her family story, never to be forgotten. This unexpected loss was unwelcomed, a dramatic detour from Amy's wish for a family that included at least two children.

In the months that followed, we explored how different she felt around other mothers who had not experienced pregnancy loss, and how this loss made her more fearful of getting pregnant again and possibly losing another child. As psychiatrists, we are told not to reveal things about ourselves lest that negatively impact the therapeutic relationship. In this case, however, I chose to share my own experience of early pregnancy loss with Amy. I wanted her to understand that, although she was feeling like no one around her could relate to what she was going through, miscarriage was a fairly common, mostly hidden experience affecting many women.

Well-intentioned people would offer up comments like, "Oh, it wasn't meant to be," or "you can always have another one." These statements were just ways to cover up their discomfort, not a way to support a grieving mom. I had felt many of the things Amy expressed in our sessions, and we united in our damaged humanity to move through her loss. A year later, Amy delivered a second child, a son, Marcus, thus completing her family and the vision she had created for herself all those years ago.

Family Building

While Amy's story had a happy ending, childlessness is a challenging reality for many women seeking to fulfill their image of family. With rates of infertility rising, many couples struggle to conceive or carry babies to term. With the promise of using reproductive-assisted technology to create families, women might delay childbearing to fulfill career aspirations. In other cases, single women preserve their eggs to be able to have a child on their own but find it difficult to decide when or whether to go through with single parenthood.

Lisa's Story

Lisa, a 43-year-old executive, had undergone egg retrieval and storage in her mid-30s. With no potential partner in sight, she had finally decided to attempt embryo transfer at the ages of 39 and 40. Unfortunately, both pregnancies had ended in the early loss of the fetus. Lisa had grown up in a single-parent household, with her mother and father having had divorced when she was 6 years old. She had one younger sister, who, at 41, was married with one child. After these two pregnancy losses, Lisa came seeking support, and with a deep wish to come to terms with her reproductive story. The older sister always felt protective and mother-like towards her younger sister, as she was often put in charge of caring for her when their mother worked late as a restaurant manager. Lisa naturally fell into the maternal nurturing role and, so envisioned that she would one day find the man of her dreams, marry, and have a family with two children, like when she and her sister were growing up.

Lack of trust was often the main cause for Lisa's intimate relationships to fall apart over the years. After Lisa's father had left her mother, she did not see her father again until she was in her mid-20s. By that time, she had been in several relationships with men that had been problematic and unsatisfying. The string of disappointing relationships made Lisa less than eager to continue dating, but at 44, she was still hoping to create a family of her own. She was a doting aunt to her sister's daughter, who was 6 years old at the time. In our work together, Lisa grew to realize that her pull towards motherhood was less about finding the perfect mate, than about her desire to care for and nurture a child. As Lisa was financially independent, she knew that she would be able to take care of a child as a single mother. She and I talked about the inherent challenges of single motherhood, and she was able to openly grieve her two early miscarriages and come to terms with the anger she felt about not being able to bear children of her own.

This was a very painful and emotional time for Lisa when a colleague suggested that she join her at an event she was organizing at a local children's home. Since Lisa loved children, she volunteered to head the carnival booth where children could receive a portrait of themselves, sketched by Lisa, who had always enjoyed drawing and painting in her free time. At one point, an 8-year-old girl named Amy came up to Lisa and asked for a portrait. As Lisa started her sketch, she began to talk to Amy, who shared a bit about her time at the children's home. Lisa learned that her mother had died of a drug overdose when Amy was 4 years old, and her father had given up his parental rights when he went to jail for selling drugs.

Amy was a quiet girl who admitted that she also liked to draw, and she and Lisa enjoyed visiting with each other that afternoon. Lisa decided that she wanted to see Amy more often and eventually explored the possibility of becoming a foster parent. After two years of being a foster mother to Amy, she became her adoptive mother. Lisa felt like a deep wound had finally healed when she chose to consider the possibility of creating a family in a different way. She was very grateful for the work she had done to understand her need to nurture a child and that she had been willing to take a chance on finding a little soulmate on her terms.

Childless by Choice

In Lisa's situation, she had finally arrived at an understanding of what she needed to feel content as related to family building. For other women, things are more complicated and their ability to realize the dream of a family is often significantly delayed or never realized. Sometimes women deliberately decide not to have children. They may struggle with being accepted and understood for their decision to remain childless. Especially in social situations, when questions turn to work and family, women who admit that they do not have children are often met with a comment like, "Oh, I'm sorry to hear that," or "I'm sure you'll have some someday." If they are comfortable enough to admit they are childless by choice, they are often met with curious looks or others questioned their choice, like it is anyone else's business but their own.

The decision to have children is highly personal, but women do experience a great degree of judgment for choosing not to reproduce. It is as if their womanhood is being questioned, as if they are not feminine enough for society. This is horribly unfair. People do not judge men for not having children the way they judge women. So this decision often entails a comprehensive exploration of where a woman is in her life journey, what her needs are, and what she is willing to be content with. For many women, our work often culminates with a true understanding of the full and glorious value of their humanity, not developing a justification of their reproductive status.

Isabella's Story

For Isabella, a talented and creative woman in her early-50s, her ability to work through a burdensome and oppressive family history served to be the most important piece of coming to peace with her decision to remain childless. Isabella was adopted in infancy by a couple who had been unable to have children of their own. She joined two other siblings, adopted from different biological families. Family life was chaotic, as Isabella described frequent arguments between her adoptive mother and father around money and her adoptive father's drinking. Her older adoptive brother and sister seemed to resent her presence and often tormented her. The home environment was emotionally cold, and Isabella did not feel comfortable much of the time growing up.

When she was 18, Isabella left home and got a job in a city about 500 miles away from her childhood home. Although she did maintain contact with her adoptive family, it was minimal and limited to holidays. When she was in her late 30s, she met a man at work who would later become her husband. With David, she felt safe, accepted, and loved, and he never pushed or questioned her distance from her adoptive family. She was fortunate that David's family was warm and welcoming but was struck by the stark contrast between this family and her own. David was an only child, having been born to his mother Anne when she was 42 years old. David's parents were in fairly good health, lived independently, and never brought up grandchildren, so starting a family was not something that Isabella and David talked about. They both enjoyed their careers, tending to their two Labradors, and relaxing together on the weekends on the family ranch.

When Isabella came to see me, it was to deal with anxiety related to public speaking. She was being required to travel and speak with groups of women about health products her company was promoting. The topic of family came up during the initial consultation when I asked if she had any children at home. She initially just replied with a short "no" and seemed eager to go on to the next question, but she then stopped when I had just nodded my head and smiled and said nothing else. She was so used to the usual questions of, "Why don't you have kids?" or "How long have you been married?" that she was surprised I was not delving deeper at this point to satisfy my curiosity of this personal part of her story.

In the initial visit, I am all about building a relationship built on trust. Although I am always alert to assessing for danger to self or others with each initial interview, I am focusing on body language, eye contact, and how someone responds to certain lines of questioning. If I feel it is important information to go after that could affect the immediate treatment recommendations, then I pursue my line of questioning. Otherwise, I give us a chance to develop a sense of comfort and ease with comes with a nod towards a respectful, gentler approach. In the case of Isabella, she was ready to delve into this topic at that moment, and so we did.

Feeling Heard

One of the most important aspects of health care, especially for women, is what we experience on the inside when we feel our health care provider is hearing us. It is a very important connection that we develop that allows us to share the most painful and difficult aspects of ourselves with another. Whether it be a visit to a gynecologist for a complaint of painful intercourse or to an internist for issues with fatigue, we need to trust our intuition about the interaction with our provider. It is critical information that needs to be heeded to afford us the most likely opportunity to get our needs met.

With health care providers becoming more stretched under the burdens of insurance requirements for proper documentation of services, burdensome hours spent trying to get prior authorizations for recommended treatments, and a lack of enough hours in the day to see a waiting room full of patients, it can feel daunting to hope for a good relationship with your doctor. It is up to us to not settle for adequate care but to seek out excellent care: the care we deserve. It is out there. It exists. And it starts with us feeling that we value ourselves enough that we are willing to go forth and do what is best for us, even if it entails effort and work. We are worth it.

In the case of Isabella, I was not the first mental health provider she had ever seen. Rather, I was one in a string of professionals she had seen growing up. Most of these childhood visits had centered around anxious, avoidant behaviors she had exhibited in her childhood. She did not feel she benefitted from these interventions because to her; they had felt forced and intrusive. That was why she had been surprised that I had not tried to rush her into a discussion of her family life with her husband as the last two therapists had. Something shifted in her at that moment, that felt like she was accepted for who she was in that moment, not judged for what she lacked. Isabella said in a later session that she was so grateful for accepting the referral from her internist to see me because she felt like she finally was where she needed to be to heal.

When you hear that from someone who comes to see you, it is validation that God has me right where He needs me and that I am blessed to be doing what I am doing. For every woman reading this book, if you are struggling with a health issue that remains unresolved, there are people out there who truly care about you and will listen, so please do not give up until you find them. This is what Isabella would say to you, and I second that. For it is in deeply acknowledging our value, that we can tap into that feminine wisdom that guides us to where we need to be at every twist and turn of our life journey. This is such a sacred and beautiful thing that I want every woman to experience. For Isabella, her journey of emotionally healing the scars of her childhood led her to me. For me, it was the beginning of a relationship that grew me as a therapist and more importantly, as a human being.

CHAPTER 5 TIPS

1. Seek support for pregnancy loss if you are still grieving. Although the loss will always be a part of your life history, getting stuck in the past will hinder the healing that needs to take place.

2. No matter what your reproductive story, be sensitive to the fact that everyone is on a unique family-building journey and what is going on your life may be vastly different from someone else's. Let's be open and embrace this diversity of experience.

3. Choosing not to have children in your life is an option that does not need to be explained or defended. It just is a choice, just like another and is your own, no matter what people may have to say about it.

4. If you are struggling to find your way through your reproductive story, find ways to explore your feelings either through journaling or talking to someone.

5. Recognize that your unique family-of-origin story will impact your vision for the future and may or may not be in sync with that of your partner. Each perspective is valid, and compromise is possible when we allow respect to rule despite the differences between our truths.

6. Trust your feminine intuition. It is a gift. If you truly listen to it, it will lead you where you need to go and out of situations you need to leave behind.

CHAPTER 6

9 to 5: Location to be Determined

Your work is to discover your work and then with all your heart to give yourself to it.

BUDDHA

Have you ever been at a social function and been asked, "So what do you do?" I know that this line of questioning is often more for the benefit of the person asking than for the person being asked. As a woman who was able to take time off from my work when my children were born, but then transitioned back into the workforce when I felt ready to do so, I have answered that question in several ways. When I replied, "I stay home with my children," I received a different response from a woman who was also staying home with her kids than from a woman who was working.

The stay-at-home mom would brighten up and feel like she had found a kindred spirit and would excitedly start to ask me my kid's ages and sexes. The woman working outside of the home would usually respond with either a gentle clucking of her tongue, "Oh, gosh, I just don't know how you do that all day!" or sometimes wistfully say, "Yeah, I wish I could stay home with my kids, but I have to work because we need the income." It has always struck me as such a fascinating reality of this age-old question; what does it mean if a woman works outside of the home, and why do we care so much?

Marci's Story

Marci, a 42-year-old lawyer, came to see me about anxiety and stress related to her work issues. She was about two months postpartum when she decided to come in for a consultation. She revealed that initially she had been excited about the prospect of staying home with her daughter, but due to complications involving her cesarean section, she was still in considerable pain and discomfort. She had planned to breastfeed her daughter but found this to be quite challenging as well, due to a combination of low milk supply and her baby's challenges with colic. Even though she and her husband could afford for her to stay home with their daughter, she called me at seven weeks after delivery asking, "Am I a bad mother because I don't want to stay home with my baby?" Marci was quite distraught over the realization that she did not enjoy this time with her newborn as much as she had thought she would and she felt that she wanted to find someone to care for her baby at home so that she could go back to work in the coming weeks.

Marci explained that her mother had been a stay-at-home mom and that even though she thought she would follow in her footsteps, she found herself thinking otherwise in the first days and weeks after delivery. Initially, she expressed that she felt like she was defective in some way, that she didn't possess the right "mommy chip" in her brain that would make wanting to stay home with her newborn the only natural and logical option. She felt the silent disapproval of both her mother and mother-in-law, both women who had stayed home to raise their children. Even her husband was not encouraging of her decision to go back to work, explaining that he had been raised by a stay-at-home mom and had turned out great. Boy, did Marci and I love his confidence in himself and his upbringing! All joking aside, though, Marci was not only grappling with the challenge of this decision, but was also feeling the pressure of her closest support network, and this just added to her sense of isolation and fed into her self-doubt.

As a woman and a physician who both stayed at home and worked outside of the home when my sons were infants and toddlers, I could relate to both sides of Marci's dilemma. The task in front of us was to thoroughly explore both possibilities, discussing the pros and cons of each, and helping Marci to develop confidence in her opinions so that she could include those closest to her in working towards a solution for the dilemma at hand. When Marci grew to truly identify with, and come to peace with what her heart and instinct were telling her, then she relaxed into the realization that she could still mother her baby in a loving and caring way, even if she went back to work. We need to allow ourselves to be still with that voice that resides in each one of us. This voice is often not tended to because of the chatter of the world's biases and other's opinions of our choices. This serves to effectively drown out what we know deep inside is our truth.

When Marci came back to see me four months later, she brought in her daughter for me to finally meet her. Although initially, she had gone back to work full-time, she grew to realize that she craved some 1:1 time with her daughter during the week and had negotiated a half day on Wednesdays that she called her "Mommy and me" time. Both her mother and mother-in-law happily rotated Saturday mornings to come to pick up the baby, so that Marci and her husband had some alone time to catch up on sleep and to have brunch together. Her husband grew to see that Marci's desire to remain active in her law practice fed her sense of self in such a way that she was able to be a more engaged and confident mother and wife. She admitted that there were challenges that came up from time to time with the current arrangement. Overall, however, she felt the permission to modify and adjust things as time went on so she could still feel at peace with her initial decision to work outside of the home.

The work with Marci highlights several key concepts that are worth repeating. First, we will not only face challenges within ourselves when making important life decisions, but we must always be aware of the subtle, and sometimes not-so-subtle opinions and influences from those in our lives. Second, we need to understand that no matter what we decide, if we have honestly and truthfully explored the available options and have chosen based on what our intuition and heart have communicated to us, then we made the best decision at that time given that set of important parameters. This means that even though we may look back at a decision 30 years later, we must let ourselves off the hook if things are not exactly like we had envisioned them to be. There is nothing more painful than to be like a fish struggling at the end of a hook. I say just let yourself off the hook and choose to be free.

Staying at Home with the Kids

For the woman who chooses to stay at home with her children, there is often a unique set of challenges that are often not discussed out loud at most cocktail parties. At least they were not openly discussed at any cocktail parties I have been to. Then again, I don't get out much. However, within the intimate confines of a group of friends, or in dialogue with a sister or mother, challenges of the decision to stay at home are often shared, and that is a good thing, in my opinion. The isolation and shame that many women experience when they are afraid to admit that it gets pretty darn lonely and exhausting to tend to a newborn, plus or minus other children home all day alone is so damaging and so unnecessary. I am not sure when this veil of secrecy started or what purpose it serves except to diminish our sense of self further and perpetuate the feeling that there must be something wrong with us because no one else is owning up to how hard it can be when you chose to be a stay-at-home mom.

During the years that I stayed home with my kids, I was remark-ably attuned to the passage of time. Honestly, before having kids, when I was running around the hospital doing consultations all day, I felt like time just flew by. When my day revolved around four main elements of baby care—feeding, diaper changes, playtime, and naptime—I felt like time had slowed to a rush-hour crawl: a painful, torturous slowness. My husband, who had recently started a new job and had wacky work hours, would almost never come home when I anticipated and prayed he would. So, when he did walk through the door, I was so relieved, I was sometimes on the verge of tears. Not because something terrible had happened in his absence, but because some days, I felt the weight of what caring for needy and very active little human beings, basically alone. It was frankly overwhelming.

Yes, I admit it. Caring for my 13-month-old son and his newborn brother was harder than doing a 36-hour general surgery shift (that was way before a cap was put on an intern's on-call training hours) but the workload felt lighter, somehow. Crazy, I know. Again, I am just acknowledging a fact out loud. I do not need anyone to judge it; just listen to it. Permitting ourselves to speak our truth, no matter what it is, without judgment from another woman is often pretty darn difficult. Knowing how vital this space of safety in expressing our true inner world, no matter how messy, raw, and real it is, is what inspires me in every encounter I have in my life's work as a coach, counselor, and woman.

Vicky's Story

Vicky, a 48-year-old mother of three, presented to my office wanting to discuss challenges she was facing in her 29-year-old marriage. She had an 18-year-old son in college, a 17-year-old high school senior, and a 6-year-old son. She had met her husband Greg in her late 20s, while she was working as a physical therapist at a local hospital where he was finishing his Internal Medicine residency. When their first child was born, she chose to leave her job, which she did not find particularly satisfying, and stay at home with the baby. Shortly after, she became pregnant again and welcomed her second child. Initially, Vicky experienced the normal stresses of raising an infant and a toddler and felt energized by the experience, as it was more personally satisfying than her physical therapy work had been. She took to her role of stay-at-home mom with great zeal, making sure home life was satisfying for her husband and their children. When she became pregnant unexpectedly at 41 and the demands of caring for an infant, as well as the needs of two active children involved in many afterschool activities, began to wear on her, she began to feel the strain of her husband's absence more acutely, and marital strife became more evident.

Initially, Vicky tried to communicate with her husband that he was spending too much time at the office and that she was having a hard time juggling everything at home with the baby and the older kids. As Greg was used to Vicky taking care of home life and not placing any significant demands on him over the last 10 years as related to the children, Greg began to feel resentful that Vicky could not "handle" things anymore. They began to bicker with each other in front of the children about everything from who would take their son to baseball practice to who would go for a late diaper run. The bickering began to erode Vicky's confidence and made her feel that her husband's lack of support indicated his lack of interest in her happiness. She began to pull away emotionally and intimately, and Greg started spending even longer hours at the office to avoid his wife. Vicky's despondency continued to grow, and she felt more and more hopeless that things would continue to deteriorate in her marriage.

Communication

Breakdowns in relationship communication come up frequently in my practice. To use a dancing analogy in Vicky's situation, she and her husband had been agreeably engaged in a tango for the first 10 plus years of their marriage. Each partner had learned their moves, Vicky tending to the children and home, and Greg providing the financial footing of their life together. They pretty much could have won *Dancing with the Stars* with their perfected tango moves. When Vicky tried to change to the salsa, Greg was unprepared for this dance and started getting frustrated with the missteps. They were stomping on each other's toes and were getting nowhere fast. Pretty soon, both Vicky and Greg stopped dancing all together. Not an uncommon scenario in relationships, but often an overwhelming pattern to change.

In Vicky and Greg's situation, we focused on several main strategies. First, we became clear on what Vicky's actual needs were about Greg's participation in home life duties. Because so much resentment had built up in this couple, Vicky's basic needs had gotten buried under the anger they were both stewing in. In the final analysis, Vicky had two main needs: wanting her husband to support her more after work so that she could attend to the needs of the kids and committing to spend time with her as a couple once a week so they could reconnect. Vicky told Greg that his willingness to help her after work and to make couple time, made her feel loved, closer to him, and appreciative of him as her partner. Greg was able to see that their conflict-resolution efforts would grow their feelings of caring and connection, and this ultimately would allow them to establish a new dance pattern that satisfied both of their needs.

Often, the conflict that arises within women, whether they are at home with children, working outside of the home, or juggling both work and home life simultaneously, stems from an incomplete understanding of our ever-evolving needs over life. I am not the same person I was, emotionally, at 20, as I am in my 40s. Most of us would agree that we all have been shaped and molded over time by the experiences, good and not so good, that we have had thus far along our life journey. What I needed emotionally as a first-time mom is different than what I need now as the mom of a teenager. What my soul needs now, years after losing my mom, is not what I needed spiritually when I was her caretaker. And what my body is telling me I need to maintain vibrancy and health now is radically different from what my 20-year-old Frito-eating and Diet Coke-drinking medical student self was thinking. When we stop to honor our ourselves and our unique needs at a particular moment in our life journey, we are more apt to be successful at making the very change that will yield the greatest result.

Society, family, and even well-meaning friends often attempt to coerce us into making a decision that is not in alignment with who we are and who we are meant to be in our life journey. I recall someone telling me the words, "Let peace be your umpire." As a person who does not follow baseball, I had to ask what the umpire does. The umpire lets the players know what the rules are and calls the shot. I then understood those words to mean that if we are choosing a path that does not give us peace within ourselves, then we are on the wrong path.

If a particular woman does not have peace about her decision, no matter what it relates to, then she needs to be guided by that inner unrest to have the courage to chart another path, even if it is viewed unfavorably or criticized by those close to her. Ultimately, aligning ourselves with our intuition and truth, and honoring that which makes us feel contented and whole is taking responsibility for creating our happiness. This is something that we should not leave up to anyone except ourselves. Have the courage to chart your unique path. You'll be able to thank yourself later.

CHAPTER 6 TIPS

1. There is no "right" way to mother. It is a personal choice and needs to be in alignment with your vision for your life and the life of your family.

2. Nothing is set in stone. Tweaking situations to adapt to the changing demands on your life is healthy and necessary.

3. Staying at home with children is hard. You do not need to go at it alone. Seek out like-minded moms and support each other as best you can. Most every mom is thinking about what you are but is just afraid to be judged about speaking it out loud.

4. Negotiate. Every relationship involves negotiation. Put the needs of all involved parties on the table and go from there. Make sure that everyone understands your feelings, wishes, and desires. If this is difficult, involve an impartial third party, like a therapist, in the negotiations.

5. Resentment with your partner is like a slow, intravenous poison drip. The anger starts as a drop, but eventually fills you to the brim and has nowhere to go except to overflow. Resentment does not happen overnight, so be aware of early-warning signs and be committed to addressing conflict early in your relationship.

6. Emotional needs change over time and through our life experiences. Honor where you are at this moment in time and acknowledge the tenacity it takes to be true to yourself, no matter what is going on in your life.

CHAPTER 7

First Comes Love,
Then Comes Marriage

*You don't need someone to complete you; you only need
someone to accept you completely.*

UNKNOWN

So, you are sitting across from your spouse/partner/significant other one morning as he or she is absent-mindedly gobbling down a bowl of Shredded Wheat while checking Facebook posts, and you are suddenly struck with a sinking feeling. "Who are you and what have you done with my lover/best friend/soulmate?" Those lovely, hair-raising, spine-tingling sexual and sensual moments that once left you hot and bothered and panting for more have faded to a very distant cobwebbed spot on your neuronal-love pathways. Is this phenomenon unique? No. Is it normal? Yes. Is this permanent? Hopefully not. The reality is, if you consult the scientific literature on lust and initial animal attraction, study after study supports the theory that there are primal drives that initiate the neuronal cascades necessary for the first phase of relationships: attraction.

Lust keeps the chase interesting and is great as long as you are competing in a sprint. If your relationship is destined to last past a few months or years, however, we need to switch our attention to marathon mode. Marathon mode is a way of looking at a relationship with longevity and ongoing mutual satisfaction in mind. Impossible, you say? Maybe not.

In my clinical practice, I see a wide range of women across the reproductive lifecycle. Because of what I see as a recurrent theme in many, but not all, relationships that have weathered the trials and tribulations of parenthood and have entered into empty-nest mode, I have altered my counseling approach towards new moms. Yes, we still discuss self-care, getting sleep while their newborn is sleeping, and pushing the stroller around the block a few times a day so as not to go stir crazy alone with their infant: the usual stuff of new motherhood.

Connection

There is another layer these initial visits that I like to introduce early on in our discussions: "Since the baby was born, when was the last time you and your spouse/partner/significant other were eyeball to eyeball, holding hands, and talking to each other about something other than the baby?" This may or may not surprise you, but most of the time, there is a sheepish look down, a shrug of the shoulders, or a flat-out, "Nope, can't remember a time like that."

Of course, this is completely understandable, given the endless array of duties required to care for an infant and often, other children. Most couples hope that there will be time for "that" later, when the kiddos are older, or they have money to pay the babysitter. I think Amelia Earhart, the first female aviator to fly solo across the Atlantic Ocean, said it well when she offered her words of wisdom: "The most effective way to do it is to do it." Not next weekend, the next anticipated solar eclipse, or when there is a "reason" to hold hands or kiss like it's Valentine's Day or a birthday, but today, now, yesterday.

Wasn't it the notable Nike campaign slogan that caught our attention with the words, "Just do it?" I am humbly suggesting, for the marathon that is most relationships, do it on a daily basis. Whether for you that is a warm hug, a wide smile, a loving glance, an encouraging text, a gentle shoulder rub, a cup of warm tea, or a romp in the sheets. Just do it for each other on a daily basis so that it is as automatic as brushing your teeth, but keeps you connected in subtle, deeper ways than you could imagine.

Getting Your Needs Met

"But why do I always have to tell him/her what I want/need?" This is the absolute most common question I am asked in my practice. My response is simple: "And the trouble is, if you don't risk anything, you risk more – Erica Jong." If we do not tell people what our needs are, then it is unrealistic to think our unique needs will be met. Romantic comedies and Harlequin romance novels have lulled us into believing that our romantic partners should be poised to read our minds, anticipate our moods, and grant us our deepest desires without us needing to utter a single word. A lovely, warm, and fuzzy concept? Absolutely! In any way based in reality? I'm afraid not. Any relationship that stands a chance of lasting into the marathon phase needs to have a space for a dialogue about needs.

Sometimes I need to close the bedroom door for 10 minutes after work to decompress and take a hot shower. I tell my husband that. When he is waking up 5 minutes before he needs to get to work and asks me to press brew on the coffee pot and make him a quick cup of joe, I say I can do that. Could he press brew all by himself? Yes. Do I need to do that? No. But the gesture creates a little space of respect and kindness that was not there a second ago and opens the possibility of reciprocation at a future date.

Don't get me wrong. After being with someone for 10, 20, or 30 years, there can be many layers of hurt, disappointment, frustration, or anger to chip away at to get back to that soft, vulnerable place inside of yourself that would even want to try to be remotely civil. I am also not suggesting you employ these strategies if you are about to sign on the dotted line of your divorce papers. I'm afraid it may be too late in that circumstance. But if there is any hope on your love horizon, and you can muster up the courage to see what can be salvaged of your bond. Then daily sprinkle little acknowledgements of each other's essential humanity (a glass of water placed on the nightstand, greeting one's partner at the door with the enthusiasm of a Labrador retriever, or a quick hand squeeze as you pass by with the laundry basket) might go a long way towards healing a broken connection. If that fails, you can always come on in for couple's therapy. There is always space on the couch for you.

As we mature into relationships and we are changing as well along the way, things that we may have overlooked about our significant other at some point in the game, may not be so tolerable anymore. It's easier to overlook these little or big annoyances when there remains an atmosphere of mutual respect and appreciation for that other person. Of course, just like with everything in life, relationships go through periods of flux. This is normal. What I see most often in my practice, that there often is not much thought given to how to grow a relationship over time.

It is kind of like tending to a plant. If you buy a plant, bring it home, and water it a few times, but then neglect it, it will slowly wither and die. I see that in many midlife relationships, whereas each person was busy focusing on kids, career, or both, there was not as much looking at each other or looking forward. Many of us assume that if things are going relatively smoothly, that the relationship is safe and on autopilot. Nothing else needs to be done. This is a disastrous way of thinking because, as we know, stuff is constantly happening in life and we need to nurture the relationship with our partner so that it not only can survive the challenging times but grow even stronger in the tough times. Sometimes all we need is a perspective shift to get things going in a better direction.

Melanie's Story

Melanie was a 52-year-old married mother of a 20-something daughter, coming in for an evaluation of her cognitive function. Since entering menopause, she had felt that she had trouble remembering where she put her car keys, what she needed to get at the grocery store, or someone's name. She was especially alarmed about this because her grandfather had supposedly had dementia, so she wanted to see if this was happening to her. We discussed the fact that estrogen does play a role in cognitive functioning and that in menopause, many women complain of similar symptoms.

Cognition

We did a simple in-office test, pencil-and-paper tests called the Mini Mental State Exam (MMSE), and the Mini-Cog to evaluate for cognitive impairment. Melanie had perfect scores on both. We also tested for correctable causes of cognitive impairment, like thyroid function, vitamin B12, and folate levels. All of these were normal. We then evaluated her currently prescribed medications to see if they could be associated with cognitive impairment, but she was not taking anything except for vitamin D3 that she was told to take when blood work revealed a low level. She was a self-described sun avoidant, most likely explaining her low D3 levels.

We then looked at her sleep, which, although she reported that she would sometimes wake up a little earlier than she would like, it did not seem to be significantly contributing to her cognitive issues. We moved on next to nutrition, which she had worked to improve over the last two years as she went through perimenopause and she had eliminated dairy and gluten from her diet and was focusing on lots of vegetables, fruits, and lean hormone-free protein. So, she seemed to be doing pretty well with her nutritional choices at this point. Finally, we got to sources of stress in her life and how she was managing with them. It was then that the floodgates opened, and Melanie revealed her biggest ongoing source of stress and frustration: her marriage.

David, a 55-year-old, had always struggled in his career. When he and Melanie first met, she had just come out of a 7-year relationship with an emotionally abusive alcoholic, and David's quiet and soft-spoken demeanor had appealed to her. Whereas her ex had been loud, unpredictable, and frightening at times, David's calm spoke to her and felt safe. When they first married, David worked for an insurance company but struggled to meet the necessary quotas to advance in the business and eventually was fired. Melanie, on the other hand, had earned an advanced degree in nursing and was the Head of Nursing of a delivery ward, well respected and admired for her managerial style.

When their daughter was born, both Melanie's and David's parents, who lived nearby, would help with childcare, so they were able to focus on their careers. The ongoing stressor, like in many couples, was financial. Whereas Melanie consistently brought home a paycheck that covered most of the family's day-to-day expenses, David routinely struggled to hold on to jobs or to contribute routinely to expenses. Initially, Melanie encouraged David to pursue opportunities that interested him, but when she realized that he was not interested in looking for another job, she began to feel more and more frustrated and resentful.

Relationship Frustration

Eventually, Melanie's frustration over David's lack of motivation to step up to the family's financial needs started to seep into various aspects of their relationship. Melanie started to pull away emotionally and physically from David, covered extra shifts at work to avoid being around him, and started complaining to friends and family about his lack of initiative. The discomfort, emotional distance, and stress level of existing in the marriage were beginning to wear on

Melanie, and she began to feel more distracted, escaping into her thoughts and contemplating getting out of the marriage. She had been interacting from time to time with a handsome and friendly Emergency Room physician over patient issues, and despite warnings from colleagues about this doctor's multiple extramarital affairs, still found herself fantasizing about him.

We pursued a course of exploring the positive and negative feelings she currently had towards David. When we discussed the negative things, I noticed that Melanie would often keep her hand clenched in a closed-fist position, as if she was holding on tightly to her anger. Although Melanie had built up quite a list of negative feelings towards David over the last few years, she was able to reflect upon many of the tender things he had done over the course of their marriage. She would smile when she recalled the special travel cups of coffee he would get up and brew for her on winter mornings. How he adored their daughter and never failed to make it to one of her high school dance recitals. And how he had helped emotionally boost her brother when he needed a place to stay after his divorce. Melanie was surprised to find herself softening gently, slowly unfolding and opening herself up again, after having felt so constricted and unyielding for the longest time towards David. She began to realize that she had let her anger rob her of the beauty of what David represented in her life and the life of her daughter, who adored her father.

The work with Melanie unfolded gently over time. We spent time looking at the differences between her personality style (organized, ambitious, hardworking, driven) and her husband's (laidback, flexible, calm, unassuming.) It took an exploration of how these differences contributed to Melanie's anger. We were able to understand that Melanie felt fearful that with their one-person income, that they would have a hard time saving enough for their retirement, as well as daily expenses at times. She was triggered by childhood memories of not having enough to eat some school mornings and a sense of overall lack that permeated her upbringing.

David had grown up with most of his needs being provided for, so he did not approach his lack of regular gainful employment as a big deal. Because Melanie had never put the two things together, that her anger towards David's lack of initiative stemmed from her fear of going without, she had resorted to yelling and getting upset with him, instead of telling him what she needed from him as a husband and father. In their situation, even after they were able to open up the lines of communication around her feelings of fear, David still was not too eager to change his ways. He felt that they would be just fine financially and still did not pursue her suggestions to work outside of the home.

This was a classic example of the theme that is repeated over and over in relationships which ultimately you only have control over your own choices and behaviors, and no one else's, especially adults. It's kind of like that Old West expression, "You can lead a horse to water, but you can't make it drink." Melanie's boatloads of helpful suggestions, pleading words, and tearful outbursts pretty much fell on deaf ears as related to her husband.

When this became quite apparent, Melanie realized she had to make a choice: shift something about how she approached this situation or continue along the same maddening path. She decided that if she created a boundary with David around getting the needs she had voiced to him met, she would need to stick with her decision, even if it was painful. Melanie recognized that it was she who was bearing the emotional brunt of their marital conflict and she was simply burned out.

When David finally showed Melanie that he had heard what she needed from him, he chose to change his behavior and give his wife what she deeply needed; to feel respected and treated like a true partner in the marriage. Ultimately, Melanie recognized that she was committed to David and had no real intentions of getting a divorce. The D-word had been thrown out there by Melanie when she had gotten to the end of her emotional rope a few times, but this had just been a desperate attempt to wake David up to the depths of her fear of an uncertain financial future. Once she recognized that these threats were quite empty on her part, she made a conscious choice to stop saying them and shifted her attention back to the one thing she ultimately could control: herself.

Although marital conflict like this is common, the outcome for a couple is quite varied. In Melanie's case, she realized that marital therapy was not the direction she wanted to head in. Instead, the next chapter of her life and marriage to David would need to take on a different flavor from what it had been for the past 23 years. The change would have to come from within. With her daughter out of college and working in a large city several hours away, Melanie grew to understand that, barring any major unforeseen financial circumstances, that her daughter was doing alright. Melanie had been saving part of her paycheck for the last 30 years of her work as a nurse, so had built up a reasonable nest egg that was slated to continue to grow over time if left undisturbed. She enjoyed her job and planned to work for another 10 years or so, further adding to the retirement pot. So really, from a financial point of view, Melanie realized that her fear of going without as she aged was not founded in reality, but represented a vestige of her childhood that she finally decided to leave behind her.

Now that Melanie had unburdened herself of this trigger for her anger towards her husband, she was able to soften once again to the good that he represented. Now, don't get me wrong; Melanie did not wake up one day with this epiphany that she would never be annoyed again with her husband. If I could bottle that magic potion, I'd be in Fiji. Nope. It was over the course of an internal shift from fear to compassion, surrender, and love. Towards David? Not so much, although Melanie's internal work certainly benefitted her hubby in the end. No, it was an internal shift focused towards herself that ultimately yielded the most lasting results for Melanie moving forward through her life.

Meditation

The first step in this was a simple homework assignment: meditate for five minutes a day for one week and report back to me if anything was different. That does not seem like a lot of time to notice change, but I like the concept of starting small so as not to overwhelm someone starting something new and then hopefully growing it out from there. So off Melanie went with her assignment to be still with herself for five minutes a day.

One week of meditation turned into one month, and five minutes eventually turned into 15, as Melanie began to notice something interesting. As a nurse on a busy OB service, she would often feel very drained by the emotional demands of her work. Laboring women needed her support, her co-workers needed to vent, and her supervisor needed her to talk to about the upcoming schedule. She felt like she was a sponge, absorbing everything around her, leaving her feeling heavy, burdened, and exhausted.

With her burgeoning meditation practice, however, Melanie began to notice that although many of the same encounters were happening, she felt lighter somehow. It was as if there had developed this little cushion of space between herself and what came at her from others, which allowed her to be ever so slightly distanced from the previous intensity of it all. It wasn't as if she didn't care anymore. Rather, she felt a greater sense of compassion for herself and for what others were experiencing too. With this compassion, came a greater sense of self-love, acceptance, and surrender into what was going on in the present moment. Although Melanie remained her driven and hardworking self, there was a new layer of softness, yielding, and a noticeable decrease in the internal struggle that had plagued her from her childhood. The little girl who never had enough had grown into the woman who had to prove to herself that she could make it on her own, until now.

Now Melanie began to appreciate more what it meant to slow down a bit, allow for moments of grace to flood her daily life, and to appreciate that there are always opportunities for growth that, unless pursued through a tiny habit, may never allow one to experience the fullness of a life examined and mindfully lived. In Melanie's case, her gift to herself became a gift to everyone she came into contact with, including her husband David, who no longer was a feared obstacle to her future happiness, but a partner she chose to enjoy more in the present. Ultimately, Melanie's willingness to embrace a different path to find a solution to her troubles freed her to live a richer, more personally satisfying life. Nothing ventured, nothing gained, I say. Amen to that!

CHAPTER 7 TIPS

1. Make an effort to sit eyeball to eyeball with your significant other on a daily basis. You will get a unique appreciation of what is going on inside of them on a deeper, soul level. A deeper truth of what is going on between you two at any point in your relationship will be revealed through this simple, daily practice.

2. You have a much better chance of getting what you want from your significant other by just telling them what you need. What you value in your relationship may not be what your partner values and this can lead to

much discord and frustration. Take the quiz at www.5lovelanguages.com to learn what ways of communicating love are most significant to you and find out what makes your significant other feel loved too.

3. Small, daily, loving gestures may not cure deep relationship hurts, but they offer opportunities to connect that may have gone by the wayside over time. Connecting regularly in some meaningful way is necessary if you want to rebuild relationship brokenness.

4. Don't wait until your midlife relationship is in crisis mode. Tend to it like you would a potted plant: water daily, or risk being left with something that is not revivable.

5. Ultimately, we only have control over our behavior, not our partner's. Trying to threaten, declare ultimatums, or otherwise, trying to manipulate your partner emotionally never really leads to lasting change on the part of the other. Focus first on what you are contributing to the dynamic and try to start the momentum of change there.

6. Committing to a regular meditation practice can help create emotional space that was not there before and may help develop more compassion for our partner's idiosyncrasies.

CHAPTER 8

The Search for Your Inner Goddess

Each time you allow your inner goddess to radiate outwards, you're the glow in the dark for someone else.

LYN THURMAN

When we truly connect with our femininity, there is a transformative power noticeable in how we connect with others and with ourselves. As a child, being the "oops!" baby after my mother had my two older sisters and then miscarried a baby boy, I felt stuck between two worlds. On the one hand, I was the youngest sister, eight years younger than my oldest sister, being dressed in adorable pastel floral print dresses my mom had made for the three of us. On the other hand, I was the tomboy, the boy my dad never had who was willing to go to the pool supply store, fishing, and mix cement while he did home- improvement projects.

Sexuality

I didn't become aware of my femininity until puberty, as it comes for most girls with our first periods, breasts, pubic hair, and of course, the school crushes. Ah, it is more than 40 years later, and I can still remember the faces and names of my Catholic School crushes.

I recall peddling furiously past their houses after school, trying to catch a glimpse of them in their backyards. Already, at the ripe old age of 12, there were the noticeable stirrings within, the external distinctions between the boys and the girls, and the quiet inner longings to be noticed and liked. These were the beginnings of the identification with our feminine essence, that delicate awareness of a vulnerability unique to being a girl, but also the power of being in possession of this feminine mystique.

I grew up in a small town with conservative and religious values. There was a subtle yet undeniable message about what it meant to be a young woman. Being respectful and obedient is what I took away from my small Pennsylvania town as I traveled far from home, by personal choice, to college in Connecticut. There, the mix of young people from all over the country was quite the invitation for an exploration of aspects of my femininity that had largely been suppressed.

I remained my cautious, conservative self for as long as I could muster but then it just happened; lust. That heady, lose your senses, and become insanely obsessed self when the object of your desire came across your radar. The only problem with lust, as we know, is that it is like a sprint. It's intense, exhausting physically and emotionally, and then it's over, either because the animal attraction has waned, you've wizened up, or the object of your lustful desire has moved on to another. Any way you slice it, those forays into discovering our inner goddess are undeniably delicious moments that seem to get buried under job deadlines, diaper changes, hot flashes, and just about anything under the sun that can affect our sexuality.

Sexual Dysfunction/Issues

Medical conditions, medications, and mental disconnections are just the tip of the iceberg when it comes to the list of inner goddess extinguishers. When it comes to feminine sexual desire as we enter midlife, I am afraid that the statistics describing the number of women truly enjoying sex are about as good as your chance of winning the Texas Mega Millions jackpot: not so hot. You are much more likely to experience a hot flash as you enter midlife than you are to truly feel hot, lusty, and bothered.

I happen to be in the field of medicine that prescribes more orgasm-killers than any other. These serotonin-based medications are either known as SSRI (Selective-Serotonin Reuptake Inhibitors) or SNRI (Serotonin-Norepinephrine Reuptake Inhibitors). They are most often prescribed to treat moderate to severe depressive and anxiety disorders. These medications can affect either sexual desire, attainment of orgasm, or both in the women who take them.

Most women who present to me feeling depressed or anxious enough to consider medication also find that their sexuality is already blunted or pushed to the back burner. These women often feel so emotionally unwell, and their daily functioning is so impaired, that they are willing to try just about any recommendation to feel better. This phase of treatment is not as much a problem as what comes later.

Once a woman has experienced symptom improvement or remission of her depressive and anxiety symptoms, there is typically a watch-and-wait period. It is during this time, after she is getting things back on track in her life, that she is still on a maintenance dose of the medication (or medications) that helped her get better. So now she is not hopeless or having panic attacks, but she is pretty much sexually numb. Her partner is super excited because he or she sees that there are more smiles, laughs, and laundry being done. Naturally, thoughts turn towards reconnecting intimately. This makes logical sense. However, on a biological and neurotransmitter level, the brain has not caught up, and this can lead to relationship conflict.

You see, even though a woman may not be clinically depressed, until we decide to taper her off of the medication, it is still sitting on the brain receptors, basically extinguishing important signal transmission on the neuronal pathways critical for awakening sexual desire. It also significantly dampens her ability to experience orgasmic pleasure. It is like flipping a switch, expecting there to be light, but instead, you still have a dark room. The woman's partner is fervently trying to get her in the mood, aroused, or screaming with an explosion of pleasure, but the expected response is blunted or non-existent. Most of the time, my patients will not admit to their partners that they are not really in the mood, or not experiencing orgasmic release. They often struggle silently, hoping that eventually, this will improve on its own. Most often, it does not.

Beth's Story

Beth, a 45-year-old graphic designer, was on a Selective-Serotonin Reuptake Inhibitor, since her first panic attack in her late 30s. She recalled the first panic attack she had as unexpected, out of the blue, and terrifying. She was driving home from a job-training weekend, when all of a sudden, she began to feel like her heart was racing, she was short of breath, felt dizzy and nauseated, and was convinced that she was dying. She was so alarmed about what was going on that she pulled into the local ER and underwent a battery of tests, including an ECG heart evaluation, cardiac enzymes, and blood test to evaluate her thyroid function. When everything had come back normal, the ER physician had told her, "This is probably anxiety. You may have just had your first panic attack." She gave her the name of a mental health clinic and discharged her.

She hoped that was going to be her first and last panic attack, but she began to experience them initially once a week, and then multiple times a month. They were distressing, annoying, and disruptive, so she finally sought help from her primary care doctor, who offered her an SSRI. The medication worked within a few weeks, and Beth felt the panic attacks were finally behind her. When she presented to me, it was to get help tapering off of the medication. Although it had helped her anxiety attacks, she had gained weight while on it and felt like it was time to try to get off of it. In my practice, if someone is on medication and could potentially get pregnant while on it, I inquire if they are sexually active. If they say yes, I ask if they are using any form of contraception. When I asked this question, Beth laughed and said, "I don't think I could get pregnant since I'm not having sex with my husband." I asked her if they were having trouble in their relationship and she replied, "The trouble is pretty much me. I don't have the desire for sex. I used to want to have sex with Mark, but now I dread it when he asks me to be intimate."

Low Libido

It turned out that Beth's low libido had not been a problem until she started on the medication for her panic attacks. Sure, there had been some lulls in their sex life over the years around the birth of their three kids, and when she was recovering from back surgery a few years ago, but otherwise, Beth had enjoyed sex with her husband. This indicated to me that we were not dealing with a primary sexual disorder, but most likely, a side effect of her panic-disorder treatment.

She had not connected the onset of her decreased desire with the initiation of medication treatment, but rather, had chalked it up to her weight gain and a diminished body image. In Beth's situation, she was hoping to get help coming off of the medication that hopefully would help get her sexual desire back on track. In many cases, however, medication-induced sexual side effects are a significant issue for people who are not ready or unable to come off of medication. In this situation, there are not many options available that have been significantly shown to improve orgasm or desire.

Within six months of tapering off of her medication, Beth was not only able to lose some of the excess weight, but she reported being able to be more aroused and to achieve orgasm when stimulated by her husband during sex. Although some people continue to have panic attacks after they taper off of medication, Beth reported only having two over that six-month period, and we prepared her to deal with this possibility by using cognitive-behavioral therapy and breathing techniques when she noticed an onset of the panic symptoms.

Beth was fortunate to be able to reclaim her sexual enjoyment because she had been prepared to come off of her medication. This experience with Beth highlighted the fact that there are many more women experiencing sexual side effects, but that health care practitioners often neglect this aspect of their health. It is also probable that many medical professionals do not discuss the possibility of sexual side effects when they initiate medication therapy because they are focused, understandably so, on improving their presenting complaint. I was guilty of this earlier in my work as well until I started asking the uncomfortable questions no one likes to ask. If you are unable to talk to your health care provider about your concerns about your sexual health, then it may be time to look for another clinician who will talk that talk with you.

Psychiatrists, especially those in Reproductive Psychiatry, which is my area of practice, tend to inquire about sexual issues routinely. There is also a growing area of Internal Medicine focused on Women's Health, and these physicians often are working with hormonal and other reproductive issues. They make a concerted effort to incorporate sexual health questionnaires into their regular evaluation of women's health.

Hypoactive Sexual Desire Disorder (HSDD)

With the recent media buzz of the release of Addyi (flibanserin), the first and only FDA-approved treatment for acquired, generalized Hypoactive Sexual Desire Disorder (HSDD) in premenopausal women, one might have thought that the pharmaceutical industry was finally shifting from developing the next pill for male-erectile dysfunction to considering female sexual health as an area of medicine warranting some funding. But the enthusiasm of the medical community was tepid at best.

For those of you who may not be familiar with Addyi, it is not, I repeat, *not* the "female Viagra." Addyi is approved for a condition called "hypoactive sexual desire disorder," which is characterized by "low sexual desire that causes marked distress or interpersonal difficulty and is not due to a coexisting medical or psychiatric condition, problems within the relationship, or the effects of a medication or other drug substance." What does this mean exactly? In my practice, many women wonder if they are having enough sex, what is the average number of times per week they should be having sex, and if it is normal not to want to have sex. As you can imagine, clear and concise answers to such questions don't exist. Why? Because human sexuality is unique to each and recommendations should be tailored to what a person wants or does not want to explore about her inner goddess.

Okay, back to Addyi. It turns out that this medication failed to gain FDA approval twice because of questions about how effective it truly was and about its side-effect profile. You cannot drink alcohol while taking Addyi and it is supposed to be taken on a regular basis, not just when you want to have sex. No alcohol to lubricate the mood and the nether parts? I don't know about you, but the last time I was out for a romantic dinner date and just had ice water with a lemon wedge was when I was 12 and crushing on my best friend's

13-year-old brother during his Confirmation dinner celebration. For those of us who are truly struggling with a chronic lack of desire for sex, completely forgoing alcohol to give regular doing of Addyi a whirl will be a tall order. There is even a "consent" form that women need to sign before I give them the prescription for Addyi that states that they swear not to mix alcohol with Addyi. Good luck with that.

Even though I can prescribe medications, more often than not, I explore ways to avoid a pill that is supposed to cure all ills. Don't get me wrong; there are many conditions that I treat in my practice that I clinically feel necessitate psychotropic medication; postpartum psychosis is one that immediately comes to mind. This is a psychiatric emergency where Mama needs to get treatment as quickly as possible, most commonly with an antipsychotic and mood stabilizer to get to feeling better. But when I am seeing someone who, for one reason or another, has lost her connection with herself, her feminine essence, and her inner goodness, we embark upon a very different kind of therapeutic journey.

I remember exactly when this mental shift occurred for me. I had just received an e-mail about a Sex and Medicine Summit, produced and hosted by Anita Teresa Boeninger, an Integrative Health and Sexuality Educator, visual and performance artist, and founder of the Embodied Femme. I learned that Anita's work revolves around increasing body-mind integration for vibrant health, creativity, and heightened somatic intelligence. I was intrigued. As a physician trained in the classic disease model of Western Medicine, I certainly had that foundation pretty much down. What I felt I was missing, however, was a way to get the women I work with more in touch with their feminine essence: their bodies.

As a psychiatrist, I do not hear the usual complaints of body ailments common to an Internal Medicine or Family Medicine practitioner. Patients don't ask me for antibiotics, painkillers, or blood-pressure medications. I do deal, however, with strained brains. For me, the brain is like the conductor of an intricate orchestra played by the rest of your body. Signals that dictate what different parts of your body are supposed to originate from this incredibly complex web of neurons, which, if not working properly, cannot instruct the rest of the body to do its business in an efficient and timely matter. Since my work is to decrease brain strain in women, and in essence, helping the conductor get back on track, I am always looking for ways to achieve this.

Psychotropic medications, if appropriate for a particular woman, can be part of the treatment plan. I always tell women, "We are not going to put all of our eggs into this one pill basket. That is unrealistic and a setup for disappointment." Rather, I say, "This medication will be just one part of a more comprehensive approach to help you regain emotional health and wellness." So, when I fortuitously came across Anita's Sex and Medicine Summit, my curiosity was immediately peaked.

Talking about Sexuality

Mind-blowing would be one way to describe the experience. I found myself listening to this wide array of passionate male and female healers, sharing their thoughts on how to reconnect with our bodies. The take-home message for clinicians like me was, "If you are not comfortable talking about and exploring your own body and sexuality, then how the heck do you think those conversations will happen with your patients?" That is right.

It's not like I am a prude or anything, but at some point in midlife, many of us put our sexuality on some high closet shelf, where it gets dusty and cobwebby. Sure, we may have sex from time to time, several times a day or never, but I'm not referring to that. Sex can be an amazing, sensual, incredible thing, and I certainly encourage all women to use it so as not to lose it in middle age. But I am talking about how one gets back in touch with what makes us truly empowered in our femininity. A woman's relationship with her sexuality affects all aspects of life from emotional well-being, creative expression, self-esteem and self-confidence, and even her relationship with food (this last point gets its own chapter altogether). So why is this so often relegated to the back shelf of our midlife closet?

Pelvic Exams

I admit that even I was a bit skeptical about how all of this talk about sex and medicine was going to translate into my clinical practice. I could not have been more wrong. So many incredible practitioners were doing innovative things, like volunteering their vaginas to medical students to talk them through doing a respectful, sensitive, and compassionate internal exam on a woman. The *At Your Cervix* documentary crew are dedicated to making pelvic exams respectful, pain-free, and empowering for women. Mindblowing! I never had an opportunity like this in my medical school training.

As a psychiatrist working with many women who have experienced sexual trauma through sexual abuse, rape, body disfigurement through disease, or medical treatment, the pelvic exam is one of the most challenging aspects of well-woman care. This very intimate exam, conducted when we are at our most vulnerable, exposed selves, can be terrifying, painful, and likely to trigger powerful memories. Even as a female medical student, though I considered myself to be a sensitive and gentle clinician, the thought that my patient might have been a victim of female trauma did not occupy the forefront of my thinking. I was hoping I could find her cervix to do the Pap smear, and that I wouldn't drop the speculum. If I had one of these amazing, nurturing, knowledgeable clinicians teaching me how to do an empowering pelvic exam way back when, boy, would I have been honored to be a student of theirs. You go, *At Your Cervix* ladies, I applaud you!

Pelvic Floor Health

This chapter would not be complete if I did not mention the words "pelvic floor." For those of you not up to date on your female anatomy, which, ironically, is many of us women, the pelvic floor consists of muscle and connective tissue that separates the pelvic cavity above from the perineal area below. The pelvic floor gives support to the bladder, intestines, and uterus (in women). Pelvic floor dysfunction affects nearly 25% of women ages 30 to 70 worldwide. The most common cause is childbirth, but other situations can lead to pelvic floor issues in midlife women. For example, being overweight, having chronic constipation, having undergone abdominal surgery, or simply aging can all lead to pelvic floor problems. Some of the symptoms seen in pelvic floor disorders include urinary or fecal incontinence, painful intercourse, or a bloated feeling in the abdomen.

Pelvic organ prolapse can occur when the connective tissues supporting the internal organs (uterus, bladder, vagina, or rectum) have been damaged, thus causing organs to fall into unusual positions within the pelvis, leading to the symptoms mentioned above. These symptoms can cause functional impairment in daily life, as women can begin to lack desire for or experience painful sex, and stop doing things they used to do before, like chores or exercising, because of the discomfort the pelvic floor pressure, discomfort, or pain is causing.

For most women with mild symptoms, treatment may start with physical therapy with a specially trained pelvic floor-physical therapist. For more severe symptoms, therapy may need to be supplemented with surgery to reconstruct the supporting pelvic structures. The most important step is not being afraid to mention these symptoms to your doctor or OB/GYN. Help is also available online if you are unable to access help for mild to moderate pelvic dysfunction. Isa Herrera, MSPT, CSCS, the founder of Renew Physical Therapy, PC in New York has studied, researched, and practiced the treatment of Pelvic Floor Dysfunction for over a decade. Her website, www.PelvicPainRelief.com, offers online pelvic courses and coaching programs for women looking to get more information and support around their pelvic floor issues. Her Female Pelvic Alchemy Program is designed to promote self-healing and offer hope to many women who have been struggling with these pelvic conditions with little support.

Sexual Trauma

One aspect of pelvic-floor dysfunction in women that does not get enough attention and discussion is the link to sexual trauma. Most of the time, a history of pelvic pain, or challenges around sex, does not come up in the typical psychiatric interview until one asks about a history of sexual trauma. Whether it is related to childhood sexual abuse, traumatic sex, or rape, many traumatized women experience chronic pelvic pain. It is well documented in medical literature that sexual abuse often has longterm impacts on women's physical health including increased risk for irritable-bowel syndrome and other gastrointestinal syndromes, overactive bladder, pelvic pain, and dyspareunia (pain during intercourse).

Among victims of sexual trauma, according to several published studies, pelvic pain is one of the most commonly reported symptoms of pelvic floor dysfunction. One theory is that these women may have a more sensitive autonomic nervous system, which gets more quickly and readily activated in response to physical reminders of trauma, thus heightening physical perceptions of pelvic discomfort and increasing the experience of pain. It is very important for all health care providers to be aware of this link between sexual trauma and pelvic pain in their patients, as interventions such as physical therapy and surgery, will be insufficient to help many women heal without an awareness of the emotional underpinnings of pelvic pain in some women.

Empowering Womens' Sensuality

Besides those incredibly dedicated women spreading the word about the Gynecological Teaching Program (GTA) in New York City and the passionate Pelvic Floor practitioners like Isa Herrera, I became equally intrigued by the work of Pamela Madsen. Her book *Shameless* is a must-read for any clinician working with and hoping to empower woman around their sexuality. Plus, it is a funny, provocative, naughty, and motivational read for every midlife woman. Pamela, I learned, is a fearless advocate for women's health and integrated sexuality. She has been described as a "force of nature," and after listening to her contribution to the Sex and Medicine Summit, I have to agree. Her dry wit, approachable, relaxed demeanor, and refreshing, frank openness struck me like the perfect storm to shower us with the tools necessary to come to a place of body acceptance and to learn how to access our erotic core.

Erotic core? I can see the eye rolling and the mildly uncomfortable shifting in your chair as you read these words. I'm with you. When I first started delving into Madsen's work, I had to fight that inner good Catholic girl who was screaming in my ear, "You are going to do what? Find your inner erotic core? Have you gone to church to pray about this?" Okay, maybe that is a bit extreme, but I know that for most of the women I see in my part of the Bible-Belt practice, thinking of one's self as a highly erotic being is not exactly fodder for regular discussion. For those of you who are rolling your eyes in the other direction, saying, "What is she talking about? I am totally in touch with my erotic core. I am woman, hear me roar!" I deeply admire, respect, and validate your inner goodness and you can skip to the next chapter. For everyone else who is not quite there yet, I invite you to join me in this journey and read on.

No matter what your amazing goddess body has been through, be it trauma, illness, disease, treatments that have left behind body changes that are very difficult to adapt to, Pamela offers women an opportunity to allow the power of pleasure to transform their lives. Besides her book, *Shameless,* Pamela runs transformational, empowering, intimate retreats for women who are wanting to heal or reconnect with their sensuality. Will getting to know the essence of our femininity make such a powerful impact on our daily life? Many would argue "yes." But again, this is a very individual, highly personal topic that not every woman is willing to explore about herself. I intend to inform women who are struggling in various areas of life, whether it be in their intimate marital relations, with body shame, or food addiction, that there are many solutions out here, and to help each woman find the one that is the best fit for her particular life journey.

As a psychiatrist, being allowed into the deepest, darkest places of a woman's soul is truly a humbling experience. It is my responsibility as a clinician to continually educate myself about the varied ways women can come to a place of healing and soul repair, controversial or not. No matter how you feel about the topic of sensuality or sexuality, help is available if this area of your life needs an overhaul. If it is something that is on your mind or something you want to work on in your life, know that there are caring and compassionate clinicians, like those of the Sex and Medicine Summit, who are passionate about helping you connect with and heal your inner goddess. It is never too late.

CHAPTER 8 TIPS

1. Treatment for mental health conditions with psychotropic medications often comes with a side of sexual dysfunction. Don't be afraid to talk to your health care provider during and after treatment about aspects of your sexuality that are giving you trouble. If your provider is uncomfortable engaging in this type of conversation, then don't settle until you find one that is.

2. Sexual health is highly individual, with different people needing varying amounts of sexual contact to feel content and desire naturally fluctuates across the lifecycle, depending on what we are dealing with emotionally, hormonally, and medically.

3. Connection to your sexual and sensual self requires a true appreciation of the mind-body connection. What goes on in your mind affects your body and vice versa. Recognizing this critical link will allow you to gain improvement in sexual functioning by taking time to consider what needs to improve in your physical health or thought life.

4. There are simple things that your OB/GYN can do to make your annual pelvic exam more comfortable. Some use a warming lamp to illuminate and warm the exposed pelvic area during the exam. Some will offer a mirror so that you can see what is going on down there. And some will talk you through the whole exam, letting you know what is happening and why. If you are dreading your pelvic exams, it may

be time to find an OB/GYN who will provide a more empowering experience.

5. You do not need to suffer silently with the common symptoms of pelvic dysfunction. Even if pelvic physical therapists in your geographical area are rare, there is a growing number of practitioners who offer comprehensive online resources to help you to heal.

6. Even if you are not willing to go searching for your radiant, sexual inner-goddess at this moment in time, know that she is there. If gently and lovingly coaxed out when you are ready, she will serve to empower you across many life domains.

CHAPTER 9

Martyrdom: Highly Overrated

After you give so much of yourself to people over the years, one day you wake up and realize that you need someone to give to you, too.

SYLVESTER MCNUTT

Martyr: *A self-sacrificing person who always puts the needs of others before one's own.*

Look into the mirror and tell me if this description sounds familiar? Do you see this behavior in yourself or maybe a loved one, friend, or coworker? Martyrdom seems to be a highly prevalent phenomenon among those with the XX chromosome pattern. When I look at a cross-section of the women I know, myself included, there are varying degrees of this behavior inherent in the average female's experience. Like with just about everything, there is a range from the light martyr to heavy-duty martyr, and just about every flavor and shade in between. Is this way of being limited to women? If you Google the word martyr, you might be surprised to find limited references to women. In the course of world history, most people achieving martyr status, ironically, were men, typically those who died or were killed because of their religious beliefs. What is wrong with this picture?

The Female Brain

Does it have to do with how the female brain is wired and how it differs from the male brain? As a physician focused on female-brain functioning, I began to wonder if anyone has looked at why certain patterns of behavior are more common among women vs. men. In my web research, I happened upon female neuropsychiatrist, Dr. Louann Brizendine, the author of the *Female Brain*. This is not your average stuffy, hard-to-ingest and digest, science-jargon-laden medical text. Rather, it is a highly readable, extremely informative, and fascinating look at the neuroscience behind the differences between masculine and feminine brain behaviors.

Okay, let's get some basic facts about the known similarities and differences between the female and male brain. Plenty of not-so-nice jokes have been disseminated over the years about feminine sugar and spice vs. male snips and snails, and I am not here to add to the debate. According to the *Female Brain*, the male and female brains have the same number of neurons, the highway system of roadways responsible for conducting vast amounts of information to and from the brain to the body parts. Yes, the male brain is slightly bigger, but that is because the neurons in the female brain are more packed together, allowing for more efficient use of space, hence a smaller total brain volume. Amazing!

Anyway, Dr. Brizendine talks about the fact that the female brain, from an evolutionary point of view, is concerned about all the things that could directly affect the well-being of the unit of people she is in contact with. This is why women tend to be more upset with unpaid bills piling up, because, in some deep recess of her brain, she views this unpaid bill as a threat to the safety and security of herself and her pack. Could this evolutionary, hormonally driven instinct to nurture and problem-solve contribute in some way to the women being more prone to fixing their relationships, often at the expense of their health and well-being? Is it purely brain-based behavior or is there something deeper going on?

I am reminded of the concept that each of us midlife women is the sum of all of our parts. By this, I mean that we arrive at this stage in our adult lives, having each weathered our stuff of childhood, successes and failures, triumphs and disappointments, tragedies and joys, and all of these things pepper how we view the world and ourselves in it. When we are born, the filter through which we see the world is more like a shiny, Windex-polished crystal-clear window. We look at amazement, awe, and wonder at discovering what this life holds.

With the passage of time, understandably so, our windowpane can get dusty and dirty, making it more difficult to see the things of life from the perspective of awe or possibility. For some of us, the window can get so dark, that there is very little opportunity for light to shine through. What happens then? I see it all the time in my clinical practice. We settle into a kind of survival mode of habit, routine, and repetition: a vicious cycle that traps many of us in self-sabotaging behaviors that contribute to our slow, painful plunge into a less joyful and satisfying life.

So, is it possible to restore our window pane to some semblance of clarity? Absolutely. Is this as easy as taking a pill that I could prescribe you? Unfortunately not. This is a gross oversimplification of an often extremely complicated, multilayered process of meeting a woman where she is emotionally and starting to sort through her past and present so she can embark upon a more personally satisfying future.

All of us are creatures of habit. I have my morning routine down pat, and it starts before my feet even contact the ground. What am I doing? Checking my e-mail? Making a to-do list for my day? Nope. I am starting my day with gratitude. I usually would reach for my phone and turn off my alarm and immediately check my e-mail or the news. I was already contributing to the brain strain that would continue to fill my day, and it was leaving me depleted, discouraged, or depressed, and I had not even brushed my teeth yet.

Emotional Crossroads

I did not come up with this shift in my well-established routine all by myself. It came from a deeper place in my life, where I was grappling with the dark, gripping, black emotions of grief. I lost my mother in 2014 after accompanying her down a slow spiral of physical decline related to treatment for a double whammy of two blood-cell cancers: CLL (chronic lymphocytic leukemia) and Non-Hodgkin's Lymphoma.

At some point in the emotional aftermath of her death, I felt myself at a crossroads in my midlife. In my mind, there were two main paths to take: despair or delight. Choosing the despair road made complete sense to me. I could continue to mourn the loss of my icon, my elegant and brilliant mother, my best friend, my staunchest supporter, and defender. That path was a no-brainer. Because in continuing to clothe myself in the cloak of grief, I was spared the necessity of looking at what was not working in my life now that my mom was gone. Being a psychiatrist, however, even I knew that this road was not going to allow me to come closer to becoming the woman I was meant to be now that my mom's daily presence and guidance had been extinguished through her death.

Delight, the other path, was for me a radical divergence from what is expected after the death of a dearly loved one. But I had this nagging feeling that eventually culminated in a dream that finally pushed me to pursue this road instead. After my mom died, I was secretly disappointed that I was not able to dream about her. I thought that meant that we did not share as deep a bond as I thought we had or that somehow, I did not love her as much as I thought I did, or some other version of a highly irrational, grief-driven, guilt-ridden daughter-syndrome.

As far as I knew, this state of mind was not yet a diagnosable psychiatric condition, just a manifestation of a broken and dejected heart. And then she came to me in a dream. I had just walked into the downstairs bedroom to check on her, expecting to see her resting in the bed. She had pretty much taken to spending most of her day in bed or on the couch, to which she would creep slowly with the assistance of her walker. Her physical energy had gotten to an all-time low, and she feared falling again. When I entered the bedroom, I was taken aback by the sight of her wearing one of the brightly colored tank tops she would speed-walk in before she got sick, standing in the room, lifting a pair of 5-pound blue hand-weights. I immediately shouted, "Mom, what are you doing out of bed?! You're going to fall or get hurt!" She just turned her head to look at me, smiled, and said, "You don't have to worry about me; I'm going to be just fine." And poof, she was gone.

I woke up the next morning excitedly telling everyone who would listen that my mom had come to me in a dream. It was not until I sat and replayed her words over and over in my head that I got it. My mom, whom I only dreamt of once since her death, essentially told me she was okay and for me not to choose the despair path. And since, even in midlife, I always listened to my mother, I decided to listen to her one last time and make a conscious effort to choose delight.

The process of caring for my mother during her illness, and in grieving her absence from my life, served as an essential catalyst in my life. There were so many moments over the years of her illness that I felt myself buckling under the enormity of her pain and human suffering. The weight of her increasing physical and emotional demands on me as her primary caretaker, and the flashes of anger that I experienced because I was losing my strong, fearless mother to this monster known as cancer impacted me in powerful ways. I found myself relating to the women coming to see me with their unique life challenges in a transformed way. I experienced a radical therapeutic shift that helped me to understand that all of us women are joined in our essential humanity. That, no matter what the particular challenge each one of us face, we are all united through our moments of human suffering.

Life is hard. Each one of us suffers. Understanding that some-times the most important thing that we can do for each other, for a friend, a family member, a coworker, or even a stranger is to serve as a vessel to hold and just acknowledge that sorrow and suffering instead of trying to push them away, ignore them, or immediately try to fix them. In learning to acknowledge feelings without rushing to judge or criticize them, we can unburden ourselves from the need to be constantly doing and allow us to be okay with being still and fully present to the reality of what each of us is dealing with in a given moment. That is true emotional freedom if you permit yourself to cultivate this different way of looking at life and how you choose to live it.

How can we get to this place of shifting ourselves from martyr-dom to a place of emotional willingness to make peace with the past, and look at what we can start to do differently in the present to create a different future for ourselves? I am, again, reminded of a quote by a leader in mindfulness meditation, Jon Kabat-Zinn, that says, "As long as you are breathing, there is more right with you than wrong with you, no matter what is wrong." For me, that means that as long as she is alive, no matter what the circumstances that have led a particular woman to seek consultation with me, we already are at a huge advantage. It is my job to help her acknowledge and verbalize all that represents her lovely, true feminine essence, her beauty, soul, and spirit, which may have gotten buried under the pain, sorrow, disappointment, trauma, or loss inherent in a life lived. Again, if you are living your life focusing on the happiness of others at the expense of your own, I am certain that there is a considerable amount of denial of who you are as a woman and a human being. There is an even greater deal of unhappiness that needs to be looked at with eyes of curiosity, rather than self-criticism or blame.

Marlene's Story

Marlene, a 51-year-old respiratory technician, presented to me for an evaluation of her depressive and anxiety symptoms. The first thing she wanted to make clear to me was that she was a "worrier." But not only was she a worrier, but her mother had been a worrier, and even her sweet maternal grandmother had been a worrier. This represented, for Marlene, a family history steeped in worry, something that she identified with and something she repeated to me several times throughout that first encounter.

I sometimes think of this as the "generational curse" moment. Although we are taught during our psychiatry training to always inquire about a family history of mental health conditions, what that questioning reveals, and the meaning behind that history, is very individual. Some women mention it in passing like you would mention a medication allergy. But some women, like Marlene, have attached a significant amount of meaning to this familial mental-health lineage and this impacts not only how they feel about themselves, but also can influence their condition.

Working with our Thought Life

I think we all can acknowledge that thoughts are powerful things. Understanding of the power of our thinking has led, over the years, to the development of various psychotherapeutic treatment modalities, like CBT (Cognitive-Behavioral Therapy), which has been validated in many studies to be as effective in treating depressive symptoms in certain cases as a medical intervention. As a pretty darn conservative psychiatrist, I love that there are situations where I can say, "Hey, let's try to tweak a couple of things in your daily routine: sleep habits, food choices, exercise, adding meditation or other forms of spirituality, and work on your thoughts first, instead of jumping to medication. What do you say?"

In most instances, patients welcome this approach, so that's what we pursue first, being mindful to monitor closely for any significant worsening of symptoms or functioning. The lifestyle changes yield many benefits, including improved sleep quality, weight and stress reduction, and overall health improvement. But the willingness to look at how one's thoughts are impacting day-to-day life can be even more powerful, and yield lasting positive results moving forward.

In Marlene's situation, she had spent her entire adult life under the critical eye and tongue of her mother and grandmother. We were both able to agree upon the fact that they were inherently decent people, but both were stuck with a way of relating to people that had pretty much gotten passed down from generation to generation in their family line. Marlene, raising her children, had done what her female role models had done: mainly suppressing her feelings and needs to care for her family, resulting in a slew of debilitating anxiety and depressive symptoms over the years.

This case of martyrdom stemmed from a learned pattern of behavior that she had seen her mother model and had adopted as her own. It was not until recently that Marlene began to struggle. The drinking, a form of self-medication, that had initially helped calm her was now escalating, and she admitted that she had driven while under the influence on several occasions. She was plagued by a lowered sense of self, as she continued to tolerate the barrages of critical comments that would come from her mother about her parenting and her appearance.

Marlene felt that the only way to have the love of those around her was to do until she could do no more, working until her rheumatoid arthritis flared up in her hands to the point that she would cry while attempting to cook dinner or clean the house. She was afraid to ask for help from her children or husband because she was afraid to anger them and risk losing their approval, as it had been during her childhood with her mother. Marlene was never thin enough, talented enough, or worked hard enough. It was a legacy of "never enough" that had haunted her for as long as she could remember.

"Why now?" I asked during that first meeting together. "I feel like I'm sinking and even if I reach out for help from my family, I'm not sure they will want to help me," Marlene replied. This cognition was, unfortunately, partially based in reality. In the past, when her arthritis was acting up, and she knew she shouldn't push herself physically, she tried telling her husband or sons that she couldn't make dinner or take them to sports practice. Her explanation was often met with disdain, disapproving words or facial expressions, and that would immediately trigger familiar childhood feelings of being not being up to par with her mom's expectations. This flood of negative self-talk would cause her to push through her pain and start making the meal, thus temporarily restoring harmony to her home.

The problem was that with each instance of pushing aside her basic needs of self-care and her version of martyrdom, she was fueling her sense of despair that drove her to increase her secretive drinking. The final straw was when she dropped off her niece one morning at daycare and the teacher, who she had been friends with since elementary school, pulled her aside and said she smelled alcohol on her breath. Marlene said she just broke down sobbing and cried for a good half hour. When she had finally purged herself of this emotional burden, she said this secret had finally come to light for a reason, and she felt compelled, even driven, as if spiritually, not to let the darkness overshadow her again. It was that day she called her friend, who gave her my name and number. The rest is history.

Although Marlene and I worked together for about half a year, we chose to spend the majority of time focusing on the "What now?" instead of the "Why?" of the past. Although we did spend some time exploring and accepting the truths of her upbringing, Marlene was ready to focus on specific strategies for moving her life forward. She was very clear about the fact that, although she loved her mother, she didn't like how she treated her. Marlene understood that, as a child, she did not have much choice about how her mom behaved towards her. As an adult woman, the reality could be quite different.

We discussed the fact that the same principle applied to her husband and four sons. She quickly learned that her self-sacrificing ways were not something anyone in her family was eager to give up. They had grown used to having Marlene responding to their every request, and initially, her biggest fear came true when she started finally asking something of them in return. Major pushback, in the form of poor attitudes and anger, often pushed her to her deepest limits. The difference now was that she was not alone. Marlene had someone on this painful journey with her who was not afraid to walk with her through the pain, tears, and fear. She stopped numbing these emotions with alcohol because she knew she could fully discharge the raw, messy, terrifying reality of what she was attempting to tear down with me and I wouldn't turn away or withdraw my caring and concern.

Much of what this relationship with Marlene taught me was something that I have been beginning to understand about psychiatry over the course of my career: that this field of medicine is special, unique, and precious. If you are a practitioner of a healing art, treat it as such. For Marlene, it was not about getting a pill to treat her emotional ill, but about embarking on a journey which finally connected her to her true self. She was able to see herself, not just as a daughter, mother, or wife, but as a woman deserving of self-love and the respect and reciprocity of relationship that she had never felt worthy of demanding for herself.

Even though our formal work together eventually came to a mutual close, our paths have crossed periodically over the years. By now, her children have graduated and moved out of the house. She remains married to her husband. Her mother passed away, but not before she had figured out what she was able to tolerate and finally accept her mom's shortcomings. I remember one time, seeing her in passing at the bookstore; she smiled at me and said, "What I gave to others over the years, I do not regret, but now it's okay to check in with myself before saying another 'yes.' I am worth it."

Many of us can relate to some aspect of Marlene's journey. As midlife women, we often feel pressured to do more than what we know is healthy, physically and emotionally. I have certainly been guilty of this myself. I hope that we never lose ourselves in all of the daily doing, that we allow ourselves moments of self-reflection. I agree that sometimes all the doing is just that: getting things done, but sometimes it simply serves to distract us from really being honest with ourselves about tending to soul wounds. We all have them—soul wounds—some greater and some smaller. Just look around you. Each woman you see is carrying an inner reminder of something significant from her life journey thus far, but it is usually hidden from view.

Always remember that you are not alone in this truth. Never give up on tending to that special part of you that makes you uniquely you: your soul. You are worth that and so much more. Know that, like Marlene, there is someone out there to share your unique journey with if you are willing to take that first step of faith.

CHAPTER 9 TIPS

1. Be honest with yourself about what life expe-
    riences have led to the filter through which
    you see life get tainted and work to identify
    what changes you could make to start to see
    things more clearly and experience life more
    authentically.

2. Life does go in the direction of our thoughts. It
    is a choice we make. If we aim our thought-life
    towards possibility and positivity, we are more
    likely to steer our emotional health up rather
    than down.

3. The toughest things we go through have the
    potential to crush us but can also serve as the
    biggest catalysts for change.

4. Each day we are alive is like a rebirth. Our
    perspective and past experiences can limit
    the potential of each day. In choosing to be
    curious and open towards possibility rather
    than shut-down and constricted in fear, we
    create within ourselves space for more open-
    ness and change.

5. You have the power to accept or reject what
    has been passed down to you. Lean in towards
    that which resonates deeply with you and do
    not be afraid to rewrite history. You have this
    one life, so try to live it as authentically as you
    can.

6. Tending to your soul is as important as, (if not
    more so), tending to your physical self. If you
    are still carrying soul wounds from the past

that are tainting your present, think about what steps you might need to take to clear out the negativity that is holding you back from living the life you deserve to live.

CHAPTER 10

Food: A Steadfast Friend or Foe

Let food be thy medicine and medicine be thy food.
HIPPOCRATES

The Western world seems to be a love-hate relationship with food. We can't live without it, but we can't eat too much of it. We are blessed to live in a country where food is readily accessible, even if much of that food is not very good for us. I remember many $1 Whopper days as a budget-conscious medical resident, walking home from an overnight shift and thinking a burger would be cheap, filling, and I wouldn't have to cook: a three for one. Many $1-Whopper days later, I didn't feel so good. I was heavier (thank goodness for those surgical scrubs that you can order in larger sizes), more sluggish, and feeling pretty hypocritical.

As a medical intern, I was sitting with patients talking about how to better manage their type 2 diabetes with diet and exercise, and I was doing neither. When you are younger, you can get away with a lot more nutritionally than when you are in your 40s and beyond. At least that is what I found. I eventually got that Whopper weight off in my 20s and early 30s, but when I got into my 40s, the weight started creeping up. What is a girl to do?

Like many of you, I have purchased multiple books touting the latest and greatest diet craze to hit the *New York Times* bestseller list.

I have done the low-carb Atkins, which made me feel so dizzy and hypoglycemic, I almost passed out on a hike. I tried low fat, which, ironically, made me gain the most weight other than pregnancy. The deprivation plan, when you limit yourself to some magic number of calories per day left me feeling so irritable; my husband would hide from me.

In my 40s, I thought there had to be a better way. Being done with short-term solutions for a lifestyle problem, I started doing the research, not only for myself but for the women I see in my psychiatry practice. I knew there must be a link between what is going on nutritionally with women and symptoms classically known as depression or anxiety.

Food Choices

Most of us have experienced times in our lives when we put what we were putting into our mouths was at the lower end of the priority list, because life, bills, responsibilities, and you name it, we take care of it, were all happening at the same time and something's gotta give. For women, it is usually some aspect of our self-care. For many of us, it would be choices about our body fuel, and usually, it was not pretty. After enough Whopper meals, I, too, was feeling low energy, lack of motivation, low mood state, and was not too happy to do much of anything after work except watch television. If you don't know, those are some classic symptoms of depression. I didn't think I was depressed, but I sure felt like I was headed in that direction with how beaten down my body was feeling on a fast food diet. I wondered how many other women who were coming to see me in the office for treatment of "depression" actually had modifiable risk factors, like nutrition and lack of regular body movement, fueling these psychiatric symptoms.

As a psychiatrist, I do a lot of motivational interviewing. This is a therapeutic method that helps to find, engage, and facilitate a patient's intrinsic motivation to change behavior. This counseling approach was in part developed by psychologists Professors William R. Miller, PhD and Stephen Rollnick, PhD. I had to finally do some self-directed motivational interviewing to see why I had not yet moved towards a more self-loving approach to nutrition in my own life. Then one day, while innocently flipping through Netflix, I came upon two documentaries that changed things for me forever. The first was *Food, Inc.* by filmmaker Robert Kenner, which gave me a deeper understanding of what I had been eating and how it was being produced. This was followed by *Forks Over Knives,* a 2011 documentary by director Lee Fulkerson that explored how changing one's eating to a more plant-based approach may hold much promise in controlling, improving, or eliminating many common lifestyle and other diseases.

As a physician trained in public health, I am always looking for the latest information to support healthful, preventive strategies for my patients. It's like the phrase we all know too well; "An apple a day will keep the doctor away." You may be saying, "well, if it were just that simple." In many regards, it might be. If you look at that advice, it is simply advocating a whole food, in its natural, unprocessed form. Not a McDonald's apple pie, or a caramel apple latte from Starbucks, but a pure, unadulterated apple with all its fiber and nutrients that can do a body good, in comparison to that cinnamon apple pound cake staring at you across the table.

Julie's Story

Emotional overeating is a recurrent theme voiced by women in my practice. There may be one or several things that they are unhappy about and will turn to food to find comfort. As inexpensive, highly caloric and highly addictive foods are available 24 hours a day from your local supermarket, or drive-thru, it is no wonder that women readily seek this out as a source of instant gratification. Julie initially came to me for help with anxiety. She was a petite, highly intelligent woman in her late 50s who had launched a successful tech startup into the world, but who now was having difficulty finding her life compass.

For most of her adult life, she had split her time between her satisfying job as a successful real estate agent and being a doting aunt to her niece, Hannah. Her husband was a hedge-fund manager, extremely driven and strong-willed. Julie had spent her 29 years of marriage trying to please and appease her husband, but despite her best efforts, she eventually learned about his extramarital affair. Rick stopped the relationship when Julie found out, but Julia's trust was irrevocably broken, and she started down a slow, self-destructive path of overeating.

Once her niece left for college and Julie slowed down her real estate business to part-time because of increasing disability due to osteoarthritis, life became mainly about living with her husband, Rick. While Julie had tried to re-engage emotionally with her husband after taking time to process her feelings about his affair, she found him to be still overinvested in his work success and his frequent golf trips with business colleagues. Julie felt invisible, and her increasing weight further decreased her sense of self-worth. Julie vacillated between feelings of extreme anger and extreme longing towards her husband.

Food became a constant companion, unlike her husband, who was either busy at work or traveling out of town. Julie consulted with a dietician, lost a few pounds, but the weight would come back. It was as if Julie gave up on herself when her husband had the affair all those years ago. It was clear that she had not forgiven him for this betrayal and not forgiven herself for not being enough to keep him from going outside of their marriage. Rebuilding a sense of self became the first line of business. However, this was easier said than done. We established that she was not interested in divorcing her husband, so we turned our attention to creating a vision for her future that was more in alignment with self-love, instead of self-soothing through food.

Given a history of childhood neglect, it was very challenging for Julie, even with her career and maternal accomplishments, to truly connect with her inherent loveliness and to love herself. These are some of the most challenging moments for me in working with women who have been traumatized or neglected in childhood. It pains me so that I can see, feel, and attest to their innate worth and capacity for love, but they often cannot see or feel it themselves.

I remember asking a woman I was working with what someone might write to describe her in an obituary. To some, this may sound like a morbid and unpleasant assignment. Bear with me, it has a purpose for this story. In 15 seconds, I had managed to come up with at least 10 words to describe her: smart, funny, kind, generous, honest, faithful, loyal, beautiful, lovely, and fashionable. In that same 15 seconds, she wasn't able to come up with a single word to describe herself in a positive light. That was heartbreaking, but not uncommon for women like Julie, who have experienced betrayals from those closest to them, starting from a very young age. Many times, they chose partners in life that are also emotionally neglectful, and they fail at healing this brokenness in themselves because their partners are broken themselves. In Julie's case, her unhealthy relationship with food would not lessen its grip until she truly embraced the idea of "I am enough." There is still much work to be done, starting with mourning what will never be in her marriage through identifying a new vision for her future, grounded in a loving stance towards herself and her potential as a deeply lovable human being.

Eating Disorders in Midlife

Although Julie's situation highlights aspects of emotional overeating, other forms of disordered eating are not uncommon in midlife women. Many people mistakenly think that eating disorders, such as anorexia, are limited to young women. This, unfortunately, could not be further from the truth. Eating disorders are treatable conditions, but they require treatment and support, which is often lacking in our communities. Without a dedicated, comprehensive approach to addressing the myriad emotional underpinnings of disordered eating, it is often an isolating, lonely journey. But it does not have to be this way. Many professionals have devoted their life's work to helping countless women finally break free from the chains of anorexia and bulimia. Much of the work centers on identifying the core fear that adds daily fuel to disordered eating. Unless you can address that pivotal piece or pieces that perpetuate the eating choices, it will be an uphill battle to gain any momentum on recovery. Women are often struggling with denial about the gravity of their condition.

Midlife women typically fall into three main categories around disordered eating. First, there is a group of women who have silently and secretly struggled with an eating disorder for years without seeking treatment. Second, there is a subset of women who were treated for an eating disorder when they were younger, which has recurred. Lastly, there is a group of women who first develop an eating disorder as an adult (from eatingdisorderhope.com).

Across all of these situations, there is core insecurity and fear of feeling out of control. In the case of anorexia, compulsively managing food intake may allow for a sense of control, but most of the time, the feeling of power over the emotional stressor is short lived. Often, there is an escalation of symptoms as women engage in more intense and dangerous weight control measures. Left unchecked, eating disorders can, unfortunately, lead to premature mortality. This devastating outcome can and should be avoided, as the legacy loved ones are left with is often riddled with guilt, anger, and profound sadness.

Why do we see a growing number of midlife women struggling with various eating disorders? Early in my career, it was extremely rare to come across a midlife woman seeing treatment for disordered eating. Now, however, I am witnessing a very different landscape, and I have had to become much more attuned to the possibility of eating disorders in the women I see, as it is a cluster of symptoms that are not often volunteered. Asking each woman about her feelings around food and eating is a critical piece of the overall emotional history and should not be neglected by various practitioners. What are some triggers for disordered eating among midlife women? There are too many to list here, but some include divorce, relationship dissatisfaction, parenting issues, illness or death of loved ones, financial stressors, empty-nest challenges, fears around illness, aging and dying, and bodily changes around menopause (from Dr. Kim Dennis – eatingdisorderhope.com).

Alison's Story

Alison, a 49-year-old massage therapist, was referred to me by her primary care doctor when she had come for a visit because she had been fainting and weighed 30 pounds less than a year ago. Alison told her that she had been very stressed about starting a new massage studio and often didn't have time to eat, as she was putting in long hours at her new location. In addition to the work stress, Alison had also just lost her twin sister after a 6-month battle with ovarian cancer. She and her sister had been extremely close, and this sudden and unexpected loss had turned Alison's life upside down.

Alison felt like life was out of control, unpredictable, and scary. She admitted that she had felt so powerless watching her sister fade away right before her eyes. Even though Alison and her sister Amy had been the same age, Alison had been born first and had always been the "big" sister, protective of her younger-by-a-few-minutes sister. The fact that Amy's diagnosis came at such an advanced stage shocked the entire family, and her decline was rapid and unrelenting. When Amy died, Alison felt a part of her had died as well, and she chose to restrict her eating in an attempt to control something in a life that felt like it was completely destabilized.

Initially, the family thought that Alison's weight loss was due to grief or depression, but she was functioning at work and home, had not voiced hopelessness or thoughts of self-harm, and denied that she was depressed. Alison would find herself feeling dizzy and nearly fainting on several occasions due to restricting food and fluids, but did not admit this to anyone, even her partner, Kathy. Kathy just thought that Alison was stressed about opening her new business and had not considered that there might be something else going on with her wife.

When Alison spoke with me, it was obvious that she was minimizing her weight loss, chalking it up to stress. I inquired about any issues with disordered eating in the past, but she denied this. It became quite clear that Alison had developed a coping mechanism for all the powerlessness she had felt around her twin sister's illness and that restricting her food had made her finally feel like she had complete control over something. With her body already showing signs of strain, Alison's eating was obviously a problem and was likely to continue if she was unwilling to address what emotions were fueling her behavior.

Even though Alison felt that this way of coping was working for her, we had to undertake a thorough exploration of the evidence to the contrary, especially as related to her physical health. Much of the work we did revolved around challenging her thoughts or cognitions with a form of therapy called CBT or Cognitive-Behavioral Therapy. This is goal-oriented psychotherapy that takes a hands-on, practical approach to problem-solving. In essence, we try to change patterns of thinking or behavior that are giving people trouble in their daily lives to foster the development of healthier coping strategies. It is often most successfully used in women with bulimia and binge-eating disorders, but elements of this type of psychotherapy can be helpful in other eating disorders, especially if there is a depressive component to the symptom picture. In Alison's situation, it was apparent that she still was experiencing residual depressive symptoms related to the loss of her beloved sister. If we did not address the depression and protracted grief she was experiencing, it would be more difficult for her to break free from her patterns of restrictive eating.

A critical turning point in my work with Alison came about four months into our work together. During one particular moment, when we were discussing how she was coping at work and in her home life, Alison began to cry. The cry turned into a sob, and she pulled her legs up into her chest on the couch and tucked herself into a near fetal position. I sat quietly with her for a few moments before I gently said, "Alison, what are you feeling right now as your tears flow so openly from your soul?" She could not speak for at least 5 minutes before she whispered, "I feel guilty. I don't deserve to be here, living when Amy is gone. She deserved to have a good job, kids, a life, but instead, it's me. I don't deserve what I have in my life. If I don't eat, then maybe God will take me away too, and I can be with Amy."

Alison's guilt over being a surviving twin was leading her to fuel a passive wish to die and be reunited with her sister. We explored the fact that she did not have an active wish to die, but rather, that her grief-laden thinking had led her to believe that if she just ate less and less over time, then she would quietly pass away from malnutrition and no one would be the wiser. In time, we were able to challenge this distorted cognition by simultaneously treating her residual depressive symptoms and by completing her grief work that had not previously been adequately addressed.

Writing letters to Amy slowly became Alison's new coping strategy for difficult emotions, and she gradually began to be less restrictive with her food choices. When a family event happened that Amy wouldn't be able to attend due to her passing, Alison would compose a letter to her sister on the prettiest stationery I had ever seen and "mail it" by putting it in a big pink box she had found at the craft store. Alison attempted to cope with her feelings of guilt, by including her sister in the meaningful moments of her life. Alison's depressive symptoms were also lessening, and she was able to enjoy more things and find happiness in again in working with her massage-therapy clients. The work with Alison highlighted the fact that unearthing the cause of someone's disordered eating requires time, trust, and patience.

Toxic Thoughts

Dr. Caroline Leaf, the author of *Switch on Your Brain and Think and Eat Yourself Smart*, has written a lot about eating, covering topics such as toxic love and toxic food; the soul, stress, and sugar; and the gut/brain connection. She focuses much of her work on the concept of toxic thoughts, which she feels lead to 75% to 95% of illnesses that plague us. What we think about affects us physically and emotionally. When you think about what fuels most of our issues around food, there is often a direct line that can be drawn to our thought life. Of course, there are genetic factors implicated in the development of eating disorders, such as anorexia, but despite a genetic component, the expression of genes in an individual is certainly influenced by our environment, which includes our thoughts and life experiences.

Eating Disorder Recovery

A leading eating disorder expert and therapist who herself has recovered from anorexia nervosa, Carolyn Costin, wrote *8 Keys to Recovery From an Eating Disorder*. In the book, co-written with Gwen Schubert Grabb, a former patient of Costin's who is now a therapist herself, they share their insights on what it takes to begin the journey needed for recovery. Costin says,

> Being recovered is when a person can accept his or her natural body size and shape and no longer has a self-destructive relationship with food or exercise. When you are

recovered, food and weight take a proper perspective in your life, and what you weigh is not more important than who you are; in fact, actual numbers are of little or no importance at all. When recovered, you will not compromise your *health* or betray your soul to look a certain way, wear a certain size, or reach a certain number on a scale. When you are recovered, you do not use eating disorder behaviors to deal with, distract from, or cope with other problems.

Among the keys to recovery that Costin and Grabb outline in their book are the importance of changing your behaviors, feeling your feelings, and challenging your thoughts around food and emotions. As women who have recovered from their eating disorders and who are now dedicated to helping women in their recovery, they offer hope that there is a way out of the darkness of disordered eating.

The road back from an eating disorder, no matter what stage of life a woman is in, can be immensely challenging, but it is not hopeless or impossible. Many midlife women are suffering silently with fears that no one will understand their motivation behind their eating behaviors or their deepest fears around giving up their patterns of coping behaviors. It is in connecting with these deepest parts of shame and soul wounds that many women carry, that they can begin to feel that they are loved, lovable, and worthy of much more than this life of disordered eating.

It can be such an isolating, scary, and overwhelming place to be in your mind, but it does not have to be tackled alone. Like all of our midlife experiences, this is not a journey to be undertaken without help. If you are in need of support, compassion, and understanding, it is available. Even if support services are limited in your particular part of the world, there are many online resources available to get you started. An example is www.eatingdisordersanonymous. org, a web-based group of individuals who share their experience, strength, and hope to encourage people on their eating disorder recovery journey.

It was not until I started asking the right questions of the women I would see, that I realized that there are many midlife women using food to cope with what life has thrown at them. There is a kinder, gentler way to get emotional support at any stage of midlife; it does not have to involve food. Just being willing to contemplate what else is out there for you if you are struggling is the first step. Encouraging you, knowing that it takes tremendous courage to ask for help, but knowing that each of us is worthy of feeling at peace, not at daily war with ourselves, our bodies, and our minds.

CHAPTER 10 TIPS

1. Symptoms like low energy, decreased desire to do things you usually like to do, decreased ability to concentrate, fatigue, increased desire to nap (a condition many of us associate with depression) can be a reflection what is going on with us nutritionally and should be revamped, if possible, before starting a pharmacologic treatment for depression.

2. Triggers for emotional overeating in women are multifactorial, but highly personal and need to be thoroughly explored and healed before any real progress can be made towards losing unwanted weight.

3. Disordered eating in midlife can either represent the worsening of an eating disorder from an earlier time in life or may develop as a way to cope with difficult experiences like unexpected medical illness or relationship betrayal. Eating disorders are treatable, and recovery is possible.

4. If you are in need of a higher level of care for your eating disorder, there are many highly regarded residential programs. If your physical and emotional state can initially support outpatient work, there are resources on www.aedweb.org where you can locate an eating

disorder professional. If you are in an area of the country with limited outpatient eating-disorder providers, there are online communities that offer peer support and advice.

5. Achieving healing and wholeness from an eating disorder requires motivation, patience, and hope (Costin & Grabb).

CHAPTER 11

Trauma:
Lasting Legacy or
Time for Rebirth

The hardest thing to ever do is to reveal the naked soul to the world. However, in doing so brings healing, growth, strength, and powerful inspiration!

H.E. OLSEN

Not a day goes by where women, traumatized in one way or another, come into my life. We are all, in one way or another, the product of some traumatic event or events. No one is immune to trauma; it is woven into the fabric of every woman's life story. Most of the time, it is direct, like being sexually abused or being the victim of a crime. It can also be indirect, like sharing in the painful experience of a loved one's debilitating, life-threatening illness. As a psychiatrist and a human being, I am constantly reminded of this truth. We are all fragile in our humanity, but our ability to cope with trauma is uniquely personal and individual. A coping strategy that may work with one person will not be as effective for another. The task at hand is to meet each woman exactly where she is in her healing process and go from there. Easier said than done, but very much worth trying, I say.

To a certain degree, we women are all walking wounded. No matter what clothes or makeup we choose, no matter how "perfect" we make ourselves appear to be, we are all just trying to thrive or maybe initially to survive. Some of us pull this off better than others. No matter, it is what we women do, and we are all in this together, even if we don't always support each other as we should. In my practice, I am quick to point out the universality of the human experience to create an understanding up front that this is a healing journey that we are both embarking upon. We are sharing in pain, healing, and everything that comes in between.

Although I have never walked in the exact shoes of the person who seeks my help, I do offer the promise to respect and tenderly hold the painful wounds that trauma brings until that day when rebirth may be possible. The questions that we try to explore in the aftermath of trauma are what now and what next, as spending too much time in the "why," the initial instinct triggered in us to try to make some sense of what happened, is often a place where we get stuck. We did not choose the "why," but we can choose the "what now." Even when bad things happen, we ultimately have the power to move through the pain to a place of deep personal growth. No one is ever the same after trauma, but who we eventually allow ourselves to become is within our control.

Melanie's Story

Melanie, a 41-year-old boutique owner, was referred by her OB/GYN because she was exhibiting symptoms of depression during her first pregnancy. Melanie had never received treatment for any mental health issues in the past and stated that she had "done fine" throughout her adulthood in managing her life. In spending time together in a session, it became increasingly apparent that this life transition into first-time parenthood was causing her emotional distress, as she needed to negotiate for the first time in her life, a framework that involved not only herself but her new husband and a soon-to-be newborn son. None of the depressive symptoms that Melanie voiced impacted her day-to-day functioning in a significant way, so we chose not to treat with medication at that time. We decided to focus on what was contributing most significantly to her current life challenges. An exploration of the present soon led to the unearthing of a traumatic past.

Childhood Triggers

Melanie recalled her childhood as having been stressful, unhappy, and uncertain. The oldest of three siblings, she found that although her mother was patient and loving towards her, the attention she craved from her father was always lacking. He was emotionally distant, disinterested in what Melanie's mother and the children did, and self-absorbed. Melanie had a hard time tolerating this and recalled that she would often act out, trying to get his attention, but not even this moved him to any action that showed that he cared for her.

In her teenage years, she began to date a schoolmate she knew her parents would disapprove of, and one evening, he raped her. She never told anyone about this, not even her mother. But this violent act left a deep wound. From that day forward, Melanie felt that she could not trust any man because not even her father had cared enough to ask about what she was doing, or who she was spending time with, to try to protect her from harm. It was as if from that moment, Melanie decided that she would only be able to truly trust herself and this thinking would be reflected in the many failed relationships of her adult years. Because of the unresolved emotional wounds from her youth, she had set a trajectory for herself where she avoided emotional vulnerability at all costs. It just felt too dangerous.

When Melanie found herself pregnant unexpectedly in her 40s by a man she was casually dating, she experienced mixed feelings.

On the one hand, she was truly overjoyed to be welcoming a child into her life, but on the other hand, she felt she was sinking once again under the weight of relationship conflict. Unlike in her previous relationships, where she could press the emergency-exit button and escape a tumultuous union, now she had a child to think of. Her childhood came flooding back when she recalled that despite an imperfect union between her parents until her father's death, they had remained together initially for the sake of her and her siblings, and later because of habit.

Melanie had begun to experience both anxiety and depressive symptoms as her pregnancy advanced, as she tried to negotiate aspects of her relationship with the baby's father. She struggled with feelings of anger, frustration, and profound sadness when discussions about their future together ended in disagreements and verbal outbursts. These were not psychiatric symptoms to be medicated. Rather, they were the beginning of many self-realizations Melanie was having as she embarked upon this new chapter: married life and new parenthood.

While the stress of a newborn can shake the very foundation of a relatively strong marital union, welcoming a child into the world when a relationship has unsure footing is pretty much a recipe for conflict. Many of the strategies for self-protection that Melanie had employed in previous relationships simply did not work in her new marriage and often left her feeling distant and alienated from her husband. When her son Malcolm was born, there were even more issues to negotiate, including whether she would sell her store and stay home with the baby, or have the baby in daycare and return to work. It seemed that around every corner was a new challenge to overcome and Melanie often felt frustrated and resentful that it seemed that she was making all of the adjustments necessary to avoid conflict, while her husband continued in his relatively detached, unaffected way of life.

What Melanie was able to voice with clarity was that she wanted to have a home life that was different than that of her upbringing. Her parents did not work on improving their marriage, and they had pretty much maintained their usual patterns of behavior throughout the entire relationship; her mom was passive and accommodating, and her father was cold and controlling. Melanie's past rape trauma was also looming in the background, influencing her relationship decisions and coping style.

The motivating force for writing this different chapter of her life was this precious newborn, but also her survival and desire not to repeat the past familiar patterns she knew all too well. Although couple's therapy might have been an option, Melanie realized that even at 40, she had emotional growing to do. With that decision, she embraced the concept of learning what she needed to adjust in her decision-making. Melanie realized that she would need to have the courage to be more welcoming or accepting of a certain amount of emotional uncertainty to soften the walls she usually put up to protect herself. This, in and of itself, was a tall order because it meant challenging the core belief that she had developed to protect herself after her traumatic rape to allow a certain degree of vulnerability to surface in her relationship with her new husband. For so many years, the rape had defined how she viewed herself in relation to others, but now it was hindering any real chance at happiness in her roles as mother and wife.

Moving Through Trauma

After trauma, there is often the "why?" Why did this happen to me? Many of us can get stuck in the "why" and we never really get past that. Melanie had not gotten stuck in the "why," but rather, became frozen in the "what now?" Her "what now" was a heightened sense of protecting her future safety by never really allowing herself to depend on another for just about anything: safety and security, lasting love or warmth, or anything that makes a committed union deeply satisfying. While this strategy had allowed her to maintain a sense of safety, it also prevented her from being able to connect more deeply with others. The birth of her son allowed her to experience a deep, unconditional love towards another being that may have been the catalyst allowing her the possibility to rewrite her trauma survival script. Melanie began to recognize that unless she was willing to approach her new marriage from a different perspective, she was destined to repeat history instead of forging a new future for herself and her son.

Although Melanie found herself getting irritated by her husband's detachment, she eventually figured out that this behavior was triggering her past childhood memories of her emotionally detached father. She learned to recognize that her husband Paul, although appearing emotionally distant, cared deeply for her and their son. During a couple's session, we learned that Paul's father had also been emotionally distant with Paul's mother and his siblings but demonstrated his affection mainly through the provision of material goods. In gaining an understanding of Paul's male role model of his upbringing, Melanie was able to empathize and connect more with their similar upbringings.

Paul, like Melanie, admitted as well that he did not want to be like his father had been, but was afraid to show his emotional side to Melanie for fear that she would view him as less of a man. It was in exploring their shared vision for raising Malcolm that Melanie and Paul were able to begin to join as a couple and take more emotional risks by being more honest with each other in session and at home. For as Christopher Alexander, the author of *The Timeless Way of Being,* puts it,

> There is a myth, sometimes widespread, that a person need only do inner work [...] that a man is entirely responsible for his own problems; and that to cure himself, he need only change himself. The fact is, a person is so formed by his surroundings, that his state of harmony depends entirely on his harmony with his surroundings.

Melanie recognized that she and her husband were both working to create a greater sense of harmony in their home life. This enabled them to build an environment that was emotionally safer, healthier, and more satisfying for the whole family to grow in. Ultimately, Melanie's journey highlights the importance of being willing to consider rewriting aspects of our past that are no longer serving us in the present and hindering our potential for a vibrant future.

Trauma is so pervasive in the lives of women. In gently holding and exploring traumatic memories, we eventually understand that we can be the authors of a new chapter of our lives. I hope that we can approach each other with a more compassionate and loving stance, knowing that we have all experienced our unique traumatic challenges. In being willing to take a chance on facing the very thing we have learned to fear the most, we create the space necessary for rebirth.

Never give up on your beautiful self and remember that there is always someone willing to hold your hand on the journey towards your best self.

CHAPTER 11 TIPS

1. Trauma comes in many forms, but no one is immune to experiencing it over their lifetime. Next time you're tempted to judge someone, remember they, like you, have probably experienced some form of trauma. Practice compassion, not criticism.

2. Emerging from underneath the weight of a traumatic experience requires a great deal of courage. It will often require a significant rewriting of one's life script, the vision that we hold of our self in relation to the rest of the world. The fragmented self needs to reestablish trust within, as well as secure a new anchor in the outside world to feel stable, safe, and grounded once again.

3. Being emotionally honest with your significant other about your greatest fears and deepest wishes for your union may yield the greatest opportunities for honest growth and deeper intimacy.

4. Don't forget to ask yourself from time to time, "How's that working for you?" Dr. Phil believes it is the one question you need to ask yourself about your current situation to get what you want and need, no matter what you have been through.

5. A new vision and a renewed perspective on our future can only be achieved through an honest analysis of what the aspects of our history we should avoid repeating and what in our present is worth expanding upon.

6. If you need support on your journey of rebirth from trauma, seek help from a mentor, therapist, or friend. You need to connect with your experience in a meaningful way to gain the transformative potential necessary for lasting change.

Nothing in life is to be feared. It is only to be understood.

MARIE CURIE

CHAPTER 12

Making Room for Mom and Dad

To care for those who once cared for us is one of the highest honors.

TIA WALKER

I don't know about you, but it strikes me a lot that I don't feel like the number of blazing birthday candles that adorned my latest birthday cake. I can still conjure up, fairly quickly, I might add, memories from my childhood. In that childhood, not only was I young but my parents seemed so young too. Now, as I look at framed pictures of myself at 10 years old or so, I am staring at a version of myself as I make the stark realization that I am now my mom's age in those pictures. Just as I was growing up, my parents were growing in years right alongside me. Shocking, but true.

Sandwich Generation

Many of you may have heard the term "sandwich generation." I did not know anything about this until my son's precious teacher Mrs. Goodman gently pulled me aside one day in the school pick-up line and handed me a book. In a nutshell, it refers to being in the generation of women who, while having career demands, or children at home, are also taking care of aging parents or family members at the same time. We are the cheese between the slice of kid and parent bread slices. As you can imagine, if we're not careful, the cheese can get pretty compressed and start oozing out the sides, creating a bit of a mess.

Being a first-generation American, coming from immigrant family stock, I was raised with a very particular mantra regarding my parents' wishes for their later years. "I do not want to be in a nursing home. I want to stay at home when I am older," my mom frequently repeated as I was growing up. I don't know if this was meant to be an order I was expected to follow, but it seeped in so deeply into my psyche that it became my mantra for my how I envisioned my parents' "golden years."

Unfortunately, my mother's last few years were anything but golden. They pretty much were awful, with her quality of life drastically deteriorating over her last year to the point of her being bedridden. She had been an amazingly vibrant, brilliant, engaging, and talented woman, a fabulous retired pediatrician, and the most well-read person I knew. In her late 60s, she was diagnosed with CLL (Chronic Lymphocytic Leukemia), an indolent condition that usually does not kill you, as it is slowly progressive. My maternal grandmother had CLL as well, but a milder form and died of a stroke in her mid-80s, not directly because of the CLL.

In my mom's case, however, her CLL mutated into lymphoma and her lymph nodes started to occupy way too much space in her abdomen. Because of the unusually aggressive nature of her illness, she was offered the chance for a stem cell transplant. This procedure, given her 73 years, we were told, would not have been offered to her as an option at most prominent cancer centers because the likelihood of positive results, given her age, was slim, at best, and would likely skew their statistics in an unfavorable direction. We happened upon a local oncologist who gave her that chance, but unfortunately, her body partially rejected the transplant and that next and last year of her life was fraught with much pain, suffering, and functional decline, which ended in her death at 74 years old.

Caretaking

I bring up my mom, not because of what happened to her medically, but because of the choices, I decided to make as a member of the sandwich generation. My choice was not my own but involved dialogue and consideration of how my choice would affect my husband and children, who were 9 and 10 at the time my mom moved in with us to start her treatment. I was very fortunate to have a husband, also in the medical profession, who was a compassionate human being and did not hesitate when I asked if my mom could move in with us. My children, who had partly been raised by my mom at various times in their childhood, could have been "negatively" impacted by seeing their grandmother go through chemo, lose her hair, lose her vitality, and eventually die. I'm sure many people I know judged me for my decision, but in my mind, there was no other option. I knew what my mom wanted, and I had to make it happen for her, no matter what.

I was told to "hire someone" to help take care of her. Concerned family and friends said someone should come and bathe her. I knew my mom, and I knew that she did not want anyone seeing her at her most vulnerable other than family, so I respected that. I would sometimes pull into the garage before I got out of the car and sob. I cried buckets for my mom and myself, as I had a very hard time seeing my formerly dynamic and powerful mom turn into skin and bones right before my eyes as her body was ravaged by the post-stem cell rejection process and the high doses of steroids and other immune-modulating agents.

It was hard, those two years just before and just after her stem-cell transplant. I prayed constantly, and little glimmers of hope would sometimes appear, soon followed, however, by tragedy. She fell and broke her hip right in front of me. She flipped backward in the rehab hospital and slammed her head into the floor, on my watch. She fell again while walking with my dad and got a brain bleed. That final fall is what shifted things. Because of the location of the bleed, it made my mom detached from what was going on. There was this apathetic, hollow gaze that I noticed when she would open her eyes to be spoon fed, but the will to fight was extinguished.

She died a few days later in the hospital peacefully, with no heroic measures, and with my father and I holding her hands, talking to her. It was a shockingly calm departure from life, a stark contrast to the immense physical and emotional struggle of the last few years. My mom was finally at rest, and although I was devastatingly sad, I was relieved for her. No more pain, no more struggle. I think that in the dying process, we are sometimes so focused on preserving the life of our loved one, we forget that it's not about us, but about them.

What I appreciate so much about my parents, both physicians, is that they have communicated their wishes to me about end-of-life care and even funeral wishes, something so many of us avoid talking about. Some of us think it is easier to let the family decide about our care when were are no longer able to. Any way you slice it, there will be a time when others will decide things about your medical care, but as someone who has been down this road with my mom, I am so thankful that we sat down and talked about what her wishes were if the quality of life she desired would not be possible. Of course, nothing is ever black and white, especially when someone's life is in your hands. But it does help to have a general compass to follow in stressful and emotional times.

When things got especially difficult around my mom's illness, it was comforting to know that my father and I were respecting her wishes. My mom specifically stated, both verbally and in her health care proxy, that if her prognosis was deemed grave and there was little to no chance of regaining a decent quality of life, that she did not want to be put on life support. She would not have emotionally tolerated being bedbound in a nursing home. I knew that about her, and I wanted her exit from this life to be as dignified and honorable as possible. Her wish was to be cremated and flown to Poland, where she was laid to rest close to the rest of her family.

I talk about this journey as a member of the Sandwich Generation because I know that many of you reading this are facing, or will face, these issues at some point. My trajectory is just that, my own. I am not suggesting that you care for sick family members at home. I know that I could have benefitted from more support, as I juggled work, my children, and the responsibilities of my mom's needs. I descended into a deep place of despair several times before I realized that unless I ramped up my self-care, I would self-destruct under the stress of it all. I cannot tell you exactly when I had that realization, but it was the one that saved me. Eventually, I started going for a walk for 15 to 20 minutes once my mom was tucked in for the night, started deepening my friendships and leaning on people for emotional support, began paying more attention to what I was feeding myself and making sure I was in bed by 10 pm. These simple things, done daily, afforded me a platform from which to keep going forward, one day at a time, on this journey with my mom.

Caregiver Burnout

The phenomenon of caregiver burnout is very real, as I felt the grips of it pressing down upon me. Many books have been devoted to this important topic because although many of us have the desire to care for and help others, it, ultimately, is not sustainable long-term at the expense of our health, mental and physical.

Countless women have sat in my office on the verge of shattering under the immense untold pressures of taking care of an ill loved one. Many would say that it is selfish to think of themselves when someone they care about is struggling or suffering so. Having been on this exact journey myself, I empathized deeply with their inner emotional conflict. I was, however, compelled to examine with each one of them the ultimate usefulness of such a self-sacrificing approach. The importance of exploring this need for balance stemmed from the reality that many of these conditions affecting those we love and care about are usually not short-lived events. Most of the time, someone is undergoing treatment for a condition that takes months or even years to get through. We talk about this particular season in life as a marathon, rather than a sprint. I tell women that if they stay in sprint mode, they will burn out quickly.

Everything goes out the window in a crisis: nutrition, sleep, exercise, and eventually, sanity. I don't know about you, but I went through plenty of deprivation mode when I was pulling 36-hour on-call shifts doing my medical training and living twice in a postpartum fog where my sleep, what I was eating, and how I was taking care of myself was pretty pathetic. My 20 and 30-year-old self could handle it. Doing the same at 40+ is not pretty, and I do not recommend that for any woman, especially one who is trying to juggle work, kids, and ailing or aging family members.

Most of you will argue that there is just no time or resources or ability for this ramping up of self-care during this stress. I argue that not doing this basic caring for the caregiver maneuvers will land you in a far worse place, emotionally and physically, than if you consider the ultimate benefit to this preventive approach. This is not, I repeat, *not* selfish. It is a form of self-love and self-compassion that ultimately translates into a far more positive experience for you and your loved one.

Listen, all of us get frayed at the edges in our hyperlinked and hypercharged modern lives. It is easy to fall into the trap of thinking of this caretaking experience as just another thing one must do. Yes, it is hard, and yes, it involves tasks that need to be done, but there is a deeper, more soulful aspect to tending to another human being that often gets overlooked.

I saw how many times interactions with my mother were reduced to a rehearsed protocol of vital signs, list checking, and calculations of how many calories she had consumed. How many people stopped to tend to her heart, her fears, and her soul? How many people touched her hand, sat down at eye level instead of towering over her asking questions, or took a moment to reaffirm her value, humanity, and significance as a person? Not many, I am afraid. Don't get me wrong; as a medical professional myself, I too have had patient to-do lists a mile long when rounding on hospital floors, so I empathize with the plight of the overworked staff.

It was not until I saw my family member in that hospital bed that I realized that my role as caregiver extends past the basics of sheet changing, feeding, and giving medications. Caregiving also involves the powerful medicine of connection, appreciation, acknowledgment, and love. It is very difficult to give freely to our loved ones when we are not doing those things that foster self-love and self-caring along the way.

Elizabeth's Story

Elizabeth, a 56-year-old middle-school teacher, came after her internist referred her to me. The referring physicians simply said, "She has anxiety." He had been trying to treat her anxiety symptoms with various medications, but she continued to get worse. When she came in for the first visit, I was struck by how gaunt and tired she appeared. What started as an exploration of what brought her in to see me, quickly turned in something much deeper. She started to cry, her thin shoulders heaving with each sob. It was heartbreaking.

When Elizabeth's tears finally slowed, and she was able to talk, she simply said, "It is too much, just too much. I can't take it anymore." In mental health practice, this type of profound statement must be carefully explored because it can signal that someone is feeling overwhelmed enough that they are contemplating self-harm. There needs to be a thorough, gentle, and detailed line of questioning to assess the safety of the person sitting in front of you.

In Elizabeth's case, she vehemently denied that she was having thoughts of self-harm, but that the recent chain of events involving her aging parents had overloaded her coping mechanisms and she had just told her doctor she was "stressed and anxious." They had not explored the underlying cause of her current mental health state, but rather, had rushed into a medication fix. It wasn't until Elizabeth had discharged her emotional dam that she was ready to explore what had led to this emotional-health crisis.

Elizabeth was one of two siblings, her younger brother by three years living in another state. She had three children, one in college, one about to start college, and one a freshman in high school. She also worked fulltime as a middle-school teacher. Her parents, both in their early 80s, had been living in the home Elizabeth and her brother Rob had grown up in. Unfortunately, there had been some subtle signs of cognitive decline in her father for the past five years. Up until now, things had been relatively manageable, as her mother had been able to help keep an eye on things at home.

Elizabeth's intense symptoms of anxiety started two months ago, about a month after her mother fell and broke her hip. The doctors had decided to operate and repair the broken hip, and everyone hoped that her mom would make a full recovery. Elizabeth's mother struggled after her surgery, was unable to regain full mobility, and was experiencing a lot of pain. It became obvious that she was not able to care for Elizabeth's father anymore. Unfortunately, she was unable to get much help from her brother, who traveled out of the country regularly and was pretty much unavailable to help her with the unfolding situation with their parents.

Elizabeth felt like she was being pulled in too many directions. On one side, she had her ongoing obligations to her children, husband, and work. On the other hand, she felt overwhelmed will all of the decisions that needed to be made regarding her parents. As her father's cognitive decline had become more pronounced, and her mother was unable to transition from a wheelchair to a walker, Elizabeth was asked to consider placing her parents in a skilled-nursing facility.

Her anxiety peaked when the social worker called her about this from the rehab facility, as she felt guilt-ridden and overwhelmed by having to discuss this possibility with her mother. Elizabeth voiced that the isolation and burden she felt over this decision made her want to shut down. She was eating poorly, mainly convenience foods, to quickly feed her family so that she could go back to the rehab facility to visit her mother. She had moved her father into the downstairs office, as she did not feel it was safe to have him be alone in his home. She had enlisted the help of her daughter, who was starting community college classes and living at home to keep an eye on Grandpa while Elizabeth was at work. Elizabeth was functioning on about 4 to 5 hours of sleep and was exhausted during the day. She was slowly feeling herself unraveling and getting to the end of her rope when she called her doctor for help.

One of the biggest challenges women like Elizabeth face is that, most often, situations with aging parents arise suddenly and without warning. We live in a society that is relatively uncomfortable with discussing plans around the inevitability of aging. It is as if in not discussing plans for what do to in the event of illness, disability, or death will somehow prevent those things from happening.

End of Life Wishes

I often recommend that people read the book *Being Mortal: Medicine and What Matters in the End* by Atul Gawande. It covers topics related to end-of-life issues that no one wants to talk about, but everyone should. He takes us along with him on his father's challenging personal health journey, as well as recounting experiences with myriad patients he worked with during times of grave illness.

Dr. Gawande tries to convey that the many decisions we will make along the way during a serious medical condition should ultimately be in alignment with what our vision is for our life. He wants us to ask the hard questions and to identify the things that are most important to us: being pain-free, being able to watch television and eat ice cream, or using a wheelchair, but still able to spend quality time visiting with friends and loved ones.

The medical interventions we choose for ourselves, or as medical representatives for our loved ones, should be moving us closer to the desired functional or quality-of-life outcomes we identify. What we want at one point may differ at a later point, as a medical condition worsens or improves. In addition to exploring these difficult conversations that he undertook with his father and patients, Dr. Gawande took time to explore the evolving models of care.

For those of us who grew up with people we knew mainly going to nursing homes if the family could not care for them, Dr. Gawande presents novel models of aging in place that are cropping up in different parts of the United States. These communities are making it possible for people to live in supportive environments that offer different services, like visiting nurses, handymen to fix a broken doorknob, or grocery delivery. These services attempt to create a sense of community and are much less restrictive than a typical nursing home. People are thriving and able to age in place in most cases and report a much higher quality and enjoyment of life.

I think that this movement in care as we age is going to grow as we demand change in many sectors of life. Most of us envision a future that is significantly different than what we have seen our loved ones go through. By supporting novel models of care, we will have more options to choose from as we age.

The truth is that we all are born, and we all will die. Those are two givens in life. Most of the time, we are ill-prepared to deal with these issues that are often laden with extreme stress and high emotions. Arming ourselves with the ability to have these important discussions with loved ones when they can still participate, and voice their opinions and desires, is one of the greatest gifts we can give to those we love.

At the very least, educate yourself about these issues. Even if you face resistance from your family or friends who choose not to discuss these things with you, you are equipped with knowledge that will enable you to participate in your end-of-life wishes if you want to. Ultimately, we do not have any choice about how we come into this world. But we certainly can have a choice about how we exit. The choice can be up to you if you decide to make it.

CHAPTER 12 TIPS

1. If we shift how we choose to deal with the inevitability of aging in ourselves and our loved ones, we can have a more positive impact on how those later years look.

2. Make a commitment to yourself and to those you care about by not only taking the time to have some of your basic wishes for your future care in writing via a living will or health care proxy, but also to have conversations about your desires. Remember that no one can read your mind and ultimately, you want your wishes to be honored and carried out to the greatest extent possible.

3. Being the sole caregiver of a person with ongoing needs is a fulltime job, and don't let anyone tell you otherwise. Accept all the help you can get and recognize that nurturing yourself in the long haul of caretaking is the only way not to lose sight of the living that still needs to be happening in your life along the way.

4. If traditional settings, like assisted living or nursing homes, are not a good fit for you and or your loved ones, look for alternative, aging-in-place options. This movement is growing, and we are poised to make a great impact on the future of care in our older years if we seek out and demand novel care communities be developed.

5. Even if you have times when you feel over-whelmed by caretaking, try to incorporate at least one experience each day that brings you some joy: opening the window to hear the birds singing, going outside to breathe some fresh air, or listening to your favorite music. A simple action can cause a powerful reaction in you.

6. As John Leland, author of *Happiness is a Choice: Lessons from a Year Among the Oldest Old* puts it, "We all have influence over how we process the events of our lives. We have a choice: we can define our lives by these setbacks, or by the opportunities that are still available to us." There is always another opportunity for connection, growth, or happiness. We have to be willing to reach for it.

CHAPTER 13

Loss, Loss, and More Loss

Bad things do happen; how I respond to them defines my character and the quality of my life. I can choose to sit in perpetual sadness, immobilized by the gravity of my loss, or I can rise from the pain and treasure the most precious gift I have - life itself.

WALTER ANDERSON

Losing people we hold dear happens at every stage of life. It does not get any easier when we are older. Unfortunately, midlife for many women often coincides with the loss of a parent, spouse, or child. Having walked through the journey of the loss of my sweet mother in 2014, I was prepared for the fact that I would continue to process the losses of the women who came to heal through a shared connection. I did not set out to share what I had gone through, but it did become apparent that the experience of loss deepened our work together and thus, facilitated healing. The grief journey is so uniquely determined that one must take the universal truth of loss and go with the flow of what happens emotionally afterward. Each woman is uniquely hurting and needs her unique healing.

Melinda's Story

Melinda, a 56-year-old retired school teacher, came to me after the accidental death of her husband Matt, a 57-year-old pharmaceutical executive. Parents of 22-year-old twin sons in dental school, Melinda and Matt had been married for 24 years. Matt had always taken care of the financial aspects of the marriage, while Melinda had maintained the home and supervised their sons' lives and schooling. In the initial interview, Melinda seemed to be presenting with symptoms that were most likely related to coping with the loss of her husband three months ago, such as difficulty sleeping, feeling distracted and absentminded, and being tearful. However, there seemed to be a deeper level of emotion that was quite palpable when sitting with her. Initially, it was difficult for Melinda to admit to and verbalize that emotion, but eventually, she just blurted it out one afternoon; "I just feel so damn angry!"

The cause of Matt's death had been deemed accidental. He lost control of the car driving back from a conference and died as the result of the vehicle rollover. Anger over losing a loved one due to a freak accident was very understandable. However, this was not what Melinda's anger was immediately stemming from. In sorting through the endless paperwork and procedures that widows face upon losing their spouse (if the emotional pain of the loss was not enough), Melinda began to learn of a secretive side of her husband that she felt blindsided by. The betrayal she felt was fueling her anger and hampering her grief work. It was revealed that Matt had been using retirement funds and slowly cashing out investments over a 6-year period, essentially leaving Melinda and her two sons in a financial nightmare. The process of piecing together the details of what had been going on in her marriage over the last few years was another burden placed on an already fragile emotional platform.

Grief

Although this is not the typical grief journey I encounter in women in my practice, it highlights the potential complexity of each woman's unique journey through loss. Whereas many people unaware of the deeper layers of shock, resentment, and betrayal Melinda was facing might initially be empathic to her irritability and occasional bouts of anger, dismissing it as part of the shock of losing Matt, they might start to lose patience with her as time marched on. She remained mired in these feelings.

This highlights the fact that, as we meet people experiencing loss, and we experience it ourselves, that the greatest gift we can give is the gift of an absence of judgment. If we truly want to foster a community of supportive women around midlife's challenges, we need to remind ourselves that unless we are walking in the exact shoes of another person's grief, we have NO idea of the unique challenges they are facing. So instead of being quick to criticize a friend who is still not up for coming to book club nine months after her loss, think about sending her a note of love and encouragement instead.

While there are often resources for grieving people, they usually include more general grief counseling options, which include support for a wide array of midlife loss: the death of a parent, child, or friend. A group of widows in our Amarillo community recognized the void in support targeted specifically for widows. Cari Roach, Stephanie Moss, Deborah Andrews, and Marilee Bulls came together to form a group called Women Supporting Women. To be surrounded by women who understand what it means to lose not only a life partner, but also an after-dinner walking companion, income-tax preparer, and house handyman has been lifesaving for many women. The following is advice from Roach, Moss, Andrews, and Bulls in an article by Jason Boyett in the September 2016 edition of *Amarillo Magazine,*

What Not to Say to a Grieving Widow

A common refrain among the grieving is that friends and family—though well-meaning—often end up saying the wrong things. "People who haven't had a personal loss don't know what to say and may be uncomfortable with someone else's pain and tears," says Deborah Andrews of Hospice of the Southwest. "That's when we fall back on our clichés." While these words might seem comforting to the speaker, widows don't hear them the same way. A few phrases to avoid.

"Call me if you need me." Immediately after a death, the desire to help is welcome, but widows may feel like they are barely able to survive each day. Giving them the responsibility to ask for help only feels like yet another burden. They will likely never call. They may not even know what they need. Instead, advises Andrews, "anticipate the need and show up. Mow the yard. Bring paper towels."

"I understand how hard it is." Unless you are another woman who has lost her spouse, this statement only hurts. It's natural to try to relate to a person's grief by mentioning a parent or close family member who has died. But almost all adults will lose their parents someday. Though hard, that loss is extremely different from losing a husband. "You don't understand if you haven't been there," says Stephanie Moss.

"At least he didn't suffer." When someone is in pain, attempts to put a positive spin on death bring little solace. The grieving need time before they can begin to look for the silver lining in a storm cloud. Similarly hurtful positive statements include, "At least he's in a better place," or "At least now he's found peace."

"God doesn't give you more than you can handle." Religious encouragements like this caused Cari Roach to question her Christian faith. After her husband Kyle's death from cancer, she felt like she was falling apart. She wasn't handling *anything*. "I heard that so many times, I wanted to scream," she says. Despite its popularity, Roach points out that such a statement isn't in the Bible. While 1 Corinthians 10:13 says people won't be tempted beyond what they can bear, "temptation is not the same as suffering."

"I'm so happy you're moving on." Months or even years after the death of a spouse, many widows are still dealing with grief. They don't feel like they're moving on. They may not even want to move on. Even if the widow begins dating or remarries, she never truly leaves the pain behind. "You think you'll get over it, but you don't," says Roach. "You learn to live with it. It is a lifelong scar."

Saying nothing. "A lot of times people will say nothing because they're afraid to say the wrong thing," explains Moss. "People are afraid they will upset the widow or make them cry, but sometimes you need to shed those tears. They're healthy." She suggests a different approach; say, "tell me how you're feeling," and then listen closely to the answer. "Let them talk and don't give advice."

Though she felt alone, Cari Roach said educating herself about grief and the grieving process was one of the most helpful steps she took. She lists three books as particularly important to her understanding.

- ♀ "A Grief Observed" (C.S. Lewis)
- ♀ "When Your Soul Aches: Hope & Help for Women Who Have Lost Their Husbands" (Lois Mowday Rabey)
- ♀ "Understanding Grief: Helping Yourself Heal" (Alan D. Wolfelt, PhD)

Although such a targeted support group may not be currently available where you live, there are many online resources, or maybe you will be moved to start a support group in your area like Women Supporting Women did.

Legal and Financial Aspects of Loss

Even though one might be able to be supported through the emotional upheaval of a spouse's loss, many of my patients described feeling blindsided by the logistics and mountain of paperwork widows have to weed through after the death of a husband or partner. Because each person's situation and needs are unique, it was difficult to advise women on whom they needed to turn to deal with financial, legal, and practical challenges of widowhood. Anna Eckert Byrne, an estate law attorney, practicing in Cambridge, MA, and a widow herself, published a book on this topic. This book was many years in the making, as Byrne recognized that there was no concrete advice out there to help steer widows back on track with the logistical issues that need to be addressed after the death of a spouse. Her book, *A Widow's Guide: Your Legal and Financial Guide to Surviving the First Year*, contains a healthy mix of the spiritual and practical wisdom that was needed to help her survive and ultimately thrive in her life after death journey. As a psychiatrist wanting to offer women more than just a haven for their powerful hurt, Byrne's resource has served countless of my patients in areas a bit out of my area of expertise.

An exploration of midlife loss includes not only the loss of a spouse or partner, but also the loss of parents, children, and others dear to us. Although those of us fortunate to have had parents around as we moved through life, we learned that as we were growing, so too were they aging right along with us. When a parent gets sick, we often buckle right in and begin to accompany them on their journey. In many respects, the time that is spent in doctor's offices and hospitals, especially if the prognosis is grave, often heralds the beginning stages of the grief journey for many. I know it did for me, watching my strong and fiercely independent mother grow weaker and more dependent with each passing treatment. Even though she was still with us, we were all grieving all that she was giving up of her former life as her body yielded to the side effects of medications and therapies, robbing her of her independence.

To this day, I am in complete awe of how she handled the day-to-day changes in her functioning with such grace, never once complaining, just quietly adapting, accepting, and making peace with this unexpected twist of fate in a life healthfully and responsibly lived. My mom's passing at the age of 74 was too soon. She had, however, expressed to me early on in her diagnosis that she felt contented about the life she had lived thus far. If she lived long enough to put her affairs in order, then she would be at peace.

She lived for two years from treatment initiation, and she died peacefully, slipping away graciously and calmly, having fulfilled her ultimate wish of putting her affairs in order. Because she had been so open about the possibility of dying, she had created a space for us to honor her wishes. I recognized that she had done the work of making peace with her diagnosis and that she had given us the gift of grace so that we would be free to accompany her during her final days with the love and caring that she so deserved. I am extremely grateful for the selfless way that my mom left this Earth, with the serenity of accepting that which she could not change. I pray daily that she is at peace in heaven, watching over us like our guardian angel.

Claire's Story

Having worked with many women over the years grieving loved ones, the protracted form of grief that can be encountered during the end stages of medical illness, although comforting to some, does not always help lesson some women's anger over the loss. I had begun to work with Claire, a 53-year-old single physician, who initially presented to me for treatment of depression. Her father, who had raised her after her mother had died when she was a young teenager, developed lung cancer during our work together. A devoutly spiritual woman who had been raised by her father going to church every Sunday, she initially weathered her father's illness with a resolute spirit and an optimistic attitude. Much of her strength was based on her faith, which matched her father's.

As his condition deteriorated, Claire began to struggle with feelings of hopelessness. When her father later died, Claire felt so abandoned that she quickly became despondent. Claire began to speak to me of her anger directed squarely at God. She was shocked at how much rage she felt towards a spiritual figure that had held such an important place in her and her father's life.

After her mother had passed, her father had made it a point to take her to services every Sunday, so that Claire could feel like she was part of a community, and she had felt supported and comforted by this all her life, until now. She began to engage in risky behaviors, like doing drugs, things she told me were bad for her, but continued to engage in these and other self-destructive behaviors. It was as if she felt angry at her father for leaving her behind in the world to have to fend for herself. He was no longer her protector, her expected source of unconditional loving support, or her hero.

As the loss of her mother had occurred at such a young age, it felt as though part of Claire had just stopped growing emotionally at the time of her mom's passing; a functional state that had lasted into her adult years. Although she was a successful dermatologist, she had struggled to connect emotionally with a significant other and had remained single for most of her adult life. She simply felt content with the relationship with her father until his death turned her world upside down.

The next year was filled with much exploration of the "what now?" question. Claire and I examined both sides of her life journey since the loss of her parents. She could continue along the path of slow and deliberate self-destruction, self-harm through drinking, and a lack of solid sense of herself and her potential as a midlife woman. Or she could choose a path largely unknown and unexplored. Of course, we are creatures of habit and tend to plod along the familiar paths that we have set for ourselves. Like a comfortable pair of shoes that we wear until they are falling apart and don't want to part with, choosing to question old patterns of behavior takes a tremendous amount of courage, and hopefully, someone willing to go along for that ride.

In Claire's situation, she was pretty unwilling to part with her old ways of relating to the world and herself. Although part of her wanted a different future, it was the fear of nothing improving for her, even if she tried to change, that made her feel like it might be safer not to risk it in the first place. This was probably the biggest hurdle stopping Claire from her creating a different vision for her future: a life full of possibility and contentment. It was hard for her even to contemplate that her dear father's passing could be the very thing that would create an opening for her to pen a new life story.

The work proceeded in baby steps, focusing mainly on gently challenging her cognitions around how she viewed herself and her ability to function autonomously without the guidance of her father. Once Claire was able to verbalize the worst-case scenarios related to change, we then began to tackle each thought, one by one. Claire was instructed to perform specific tasks that she felt would demonstrate her independence. With each success, she was able to begin to see herself as a more effective, proactive, and mature person. Another layer of her confidence came in understanding that even though some of the risks she was taking in gaining a more grounded sense of herself might not work out as expected, we would explore these outcomes, guide her through the challenges, and see what emotional growth could be gained.

In the two years that we worked together, even though there were moments of crisis and substance relapse, Claire was truly gaining more solid, positive ground month by month. For me, it was really about keeping the healing momentum moving forward. I had committed myself to that. And Claire, who initially used my presence as a parental replacement for the support she used to receive from her father, eventually needed me less and less.

As she got more invested in the progress she was making, she recognized that she had a lot of potential as someone who might be able to move others through their grief. She started volunteering at a grief-support center and eventually connected emotionally with someone who had also experienced loss. They started dating. When we finally decided to part ways, Claire made a profound observation:

> "Holding on to this part of myself that felt so comfortable for so long began to suffocate me. I felt that if I didn't swim as fast and as hard as I could, that I would eventually drown. I could never do that to my parents. They always wanted more for me than I wanted for myself, until now."

Moving through loss is possible, but it is hard and requires consistent self-love, a willingness to challenge old ways of thinking, and a desire to challenge the status quo. For any of you who are experiencing loss, whether recent or protracted, know that you are not alone. The power to create beauty from the ashes of loss is within each one of us. If you are feeling stuck, know that there are caring people like Claire and others who want to see you thrive. Don't be afraid to reach out; there is a safety net that will catch you.

CHAPTER 13 TIPS

1. Losing someone we love is like losing part of ourself. We will always carry this piece of this grief with us, but we must eventually choose whether or not we want this loss to define us.

2. Supporting someone who has lost a spouse or significant other requires a different supportive skill set. Be sure to include widows in social activities that might include couples. They can always say "no, thank you," but it means a lot to know they matter to you.

3. Unless someone is stuck in grief and cannot function in their day-to-day life, be patient with their grief timeline, as it is uniquely their own.

4. If you feel you are drowning in your grief and cannot come up for air, you are not alone. There is support available. Don't hesitate to reach for it.

5. Sometimes those closest to us are not the most helpful sources of support and encouragement, as they are hurting in their own right or are afraid to bring up the loss for fear of reopening painful wounds. Have grace for yourself and those closest to you. You are all in this together, just in different ways.

6. Even as you mourn your loss, never forget that you are still living. Maybe starting to live again is the path to honor your loved one's memory. They will never be forgotten, whether you stay grounded in grief or permit yourself to live again.

CHAPTER 14

Still Standing,
Now What?

They always say that time changes things, but you actually have to change them yourself.

ANDY WARHOL,
IN *WARHOL: THE BIOGRAPHY*
BY VICTOR BOCKRIS

Although this is the final chapter of this book, I am confident that this current moment signifies the beginning of a brand-new chapter of your life story and that this will mark a period that you can become one of the best of your life. Yes, I know that for many of us, that is a tall order, as once we hit midlife, many of us feel like the energy, vitality, and enthusiasm of our younger years has tempered, if not extinguished, many of those previously held dreams, aspirations, and beliefs we were holding on to.

This is one area of my work with women that I put a great deal of emphasis on, as it tends to determine the quality of our "midlife and beyond" experience. No matter who is sitting in front of me, no matter what challenges, hurts, hurdles, or obstacles exist, I truly feel that each one of us owes it to our self to be courageous and honest with all the potential barriers that are holding us back from living a fulfilling midlife and beyond, and to do something about it.

Hurts, past mistakes, wrongs done to us, and regrets mark us and are often woven into the very fabric of how we view ourselves and others. As I reflect upon who I was 10 and 20 years ago as compared to who I am now, I can certainly say that I have changed. Mostly through the challenges I have faced in my health and caregiving, but also in navigating relationships with family and friends, I have been brought to my knees with the intensity of the sadness, struggle, and grief of difficult moments in this journey called life. When the tears finally dry up, and the emotional torrent has subsided, I find myself faced with two main options: sink or swim. Sink means allowing someone or something to continue to control my emotions and the quality of my life. Swim means to mobilize my anger (yes, anger can be used as a motivational tool if harnessed positively) or resolve that I can and must do something positive moving forward.

To be honest, I think I'm wired to swim, which is something I'm very grateful for. I hold on to that core belief that the challenges that I have gone through have the potential to grow or damage me, and that I must choose which one of those two realities to hold on to. I choose to believe that I, like each one of us, am a beautiful, albeit messy, work in progress, and that every heartache, disappointment, loss, and betrayal is part of our journey, whether we like it or not. Sink or swim: your choice. But know that a life vest is always available to you if you choose to reach for it.

Eloise's Story

Eloise, a 65-year-old mother of four, lived a life that most of us would feel contented with: a relatively new car and home, plenty saved up in retirement and investments, and good health, other than some aches and pains. Life should be rosy, right? Although she had launched four successful adults into the world and had a gaggle of adoring grandkids, life was a chronic source of discontent. When we explored how she was feeling at this point in her life, we hit upon several emotional roadblocks: anger, hurt, resentment, sorrow, fear, and hopelessness. We explored the Eloise of childhood and young adulthood and contrasted her with the Eloise of today. What was different? What had changed? What was missing?

In a rare moment during a session together where raw emotion pushed through her usually emotionally collected, intellectual veneer, tears began to well up in her eyes as she barely whispered the words, "Love. I don't believe anyone has really loved me and I don't even love myself." A deep, powerful, hidden, shame-laden truth was finally released into the universe, was no longer a thought keeping her a prisoner of her mind. I honored, held, and tolerated that forbidden truth in another woman and did not turn away, reject, or try to fix her. We just sat together in the space of my office, the machine-generated sound of soothing ocean waves washing over us, cleansing, soothing, and settling us into this revealed truth.

Vulnerability

Vulnerability in our relationships is something that many of us struggle with. Often, being honest about how we are feeling or how we are struggling feels shameful and often remains hidden even in our most intimate of relationships. Many times, we are just wanting to avoid feeling judged, even by people we consider close friends. We are afraid that we will be rejected or thought of as being damaged or defective, so we live behind a cheerful, agreeable mask, while inside, we are slowly dying.

None of us thrive as women when we live in disharmony with our true inner voice. This voice is what is meant to guide us along the path that is most in alignment with our purpose and the source of joy of being alive. Even when life has not turned out how we have hoped, dreamed, or planned it would, we still have the choice to listen to that still, small voice inside of us that will guide us towards our true purpose, no matter where we are in our midlife journey.

Soul Connection

What is your soul telling you that you need more of today? Connection with another, self-love, self-care, or pursuing a wish or dream? Ask yourself each morning, "What can I do today to bring a smile to my or another's face today?" and figure out how to make that a reality. One day at a time. Each day, permit yourself to think about what you would like to do that expands your life or connects you to something meaningful and do it. For as Robert Louis Stevenson in *An Inland Voyage* put it, "To know what you prefer, instead of humbly saying Amen to what the world tells you ought to prefer, is to have kept your soul alive."

How many of us are being held back from stepping into a rich chapter of our life experience by past hurts, shamed into believing that, as women, we need to keep these soul wounds hidden, locked away to slowly but surely erode our innate sense of self, once so pure and unblemished?

It is my mission to serve the women who seek affirmation of their true selves through the process of laying down the truths of a life lived thus far while committing the self to take ownership and authorship of the "rest of their life" narrative. I, for one, am signing up to read the first chapter of each one of your midlife and beyond memoirs, as it is only through the honest exploration of the self that we gain the courage to look at what is missing and gain the wisdom to make the rest of your life the best of your life.

Being your Own Best Friend

I have had many women at midlife and beyond say, "I don't know what I want." When they express unhappiness about the state of their relationships, health, body image, ongoing grief, or unrealized dreams, we often need to backtrack to an earlier time in their life that they remember feeling confident, happy, or content. We try to connect with the emotional state of that positive memory and slowly start to build a more solid sense of self. How do you do that when you feel that you have gotten to a point in your adult life where you feel beaten down by adversity, whether it be illness, death, betrayal, or loss? I guess I go back to the concept of what it takes to be one's own best friend. I remind women that if a friend came to them feeling downtrodden or overwhelmed, they would lovingly listen and offer care, comfort, and a safe space for healing. Why, then, is it so hard to do that for ourselves when we need restoration, hope, and renewal?

One theory is that, as women, no matter what life stage we are in, there is usually more to attend to than just ourselves. If we have a husband or partner, there are often issues related to caring for their needs, such as in illness. There can also be grandchildren or even launched children, who, as adults, are still struggling for stability and often turn to family for financial and other forms of concrete support that continue to demand our time and attention. Sometimes, we may struggle with our health issues that make looking at the "now what?" time of our lives with fear and hesitation. If some or all of these scenarios have appeared in your life, it is understandable that there may not be enough energy left over to dream and go after those dreams. However, I fervently believe those dreams are still worth going after, even if you have to start out slowly.

For example, for a woman who has just experienced the crushing loss of her husband of 30 years, once she is supported through the first years of grief work, and the reorganizing of daily financial and practical life, I might start to explore the "what now" question with her. I may ask what makes her smile, what peaks her curiosity, or what makes her soul sing. Sometimes, I get a blank stare, like how can thinking about something other than loss even be on the table for discussion. But I gently plod on. I will ask about the last thing that she felt truly excited or exhilarated about, and if I get a nibble, then I explore that further. No matter who you are, what you have been through and survived, or what you are going through at this moment in time, there is something in all of us that deserves to be taken one step further.

For Eloise, it was films. Her voracious, insatiable, and ever-demanding appetite for the cinema of all genres burned like a flame inside of her and despite everything she had experienced, remained a constant source of joy, excitement, and mystery, even in the darkest times of betrayal and loneliness. Going to the movies had both functioned as an escape from the realities of her life, while at the same time, offering her comfort that she was not alone in life's struggles. At least this was an anchor, a starting point from which to start to build a different vision for her life now that her children were grown, and her husband was still deeply pursuing his career ventures.

Eloise and I met once a week, building with each session layers of herself that would eventually form a more cohesive template for daily life. Up until this point, there had not been a mindful contemplation of how to best structure a routine that would allow Eloise to experience each day to the fullest. She often complained that she lacked the motivation to achieve goals. Eventually, we grew to understand that she did not feel truly contented because she lacked in several core fundamental aspects of physical and emotional health. We outlined the various aspects of herself that had been neglected over the years and we set about defining how attending to each of these areas would allow her to feel more balanced and mindful.

Healthier Life Choices

Her weight had been problematic for her for the last 10 years, leading to chronic joint pain and a decreased ability to enjoy being physically active. We decided to devote time to outlining daily, simple practices that she could cultivate and nurture over time, which would allow her to have a greater appreciation for what her body could do given a chance to heal and strengthen. For so much of her life, Eloise had been consumed, like many of us, with the final destination, the dramatic weight loss goal she had put in her mind. She would start off extremely motivated, lose a few pounds, but quickly lose steam as her hunger and irritability grew. We needed to shift that high-pressure mentality towards a kinder and gentler vision for herself, her health, and her vitality. For in engaging in the usual punishing methods of weight loss, based on a model of deprivation and harsh assessments of her body, Eloise was in warrior mode with herself, engaging in an unnecessary and unhelpful battle with the most important person in the world: herself.

Once we had established some basic guidelines based on a straight-forward, anti-inflammatory, whole-foods way of eating (I like Dr. Terry Wahl's food protocol www.terrywahls.com or Dr. Joel Fuhrman's nutritarian approach www.drfuhrman.com), we moved on to nurturing her physical self. For so many years, given her excess weight, Eloise had just about resigned herself to a daily existence with limited physical activity. Again, a big barrier to her motivation was this all-or-nothing mentality. She would compare herself to the neighbor going for a walk or a friend going to yoga class and would always, in her mind, fall short. This negative assessment of herself would fuel her despair and usually end with a trip through the local restaurant drive-thru. With her knee troubles, we focused on what SHE could comfortably do, not what anyone else could do. Unless Eloise decided that she was going to run her race, not anyone else's, she would always fall short and feel shackled to unrealistic expectations that she would not be able to live up to. This would again fuel her disappointment and sense of failure in herself.

Even at 65 years old, we had to work a bit to develop a more secure sense of self, so that Eloise embraced the concept of doing what's best for HER, not anyone else, given her current physical limitations. In Eloise's situation, we decided on a weekly water aerobics class. We also decided that she would start a meditation practice that consisted of her opening the Calm app on her smartphone and just spending 5 minutes a day breathing in and out through her nose, activating the calming, centering, parasympathetic nervous system along the way.

Over the next month, 5 minutes turned into 10, and six months later, into a 20-minute meditation practice that allowed Eloise to become much more in tune with where her thought life tended to wander. Her new awareness of the negative self-talk that had plagued much of her life had only become possible through cultivating this practice of really paying attention to the flavor of her inner dialogue. Once she had developed a true understanding of how damaging this was to her soul, she was poised to use this newfound knowledge to move forward with intention, instead of the usual course of mindless repetition that had consumed the last few years of her life.

After we had solidified a plan of action for a daily practice of nurturing her physical body, we moved on to another area of disconnect: her relationships with others. Although Eloise had several people in her inner circle, each relationship was conflicted and often served as a source of recurrent pain. This would often lead to anger and resentment, as she felt that she still often prioritized their needs at the expense of her own. We talked about the fact that as human beings, we have an inherent need to connect with others to feel grounded. All of us, even the tiniest of newborns, need to have a connection to survive and, ultimately, thrive.

The challenges that often arise in our adult attempts at connection are that they are often based, to some extent, on our childhood relationships and experiences with the adults who were responsible for our care and safety. The sad truth is that many adults are walking wounded. Many of us are grown-ups who, to this day, struggle with the remnants of soul wounds inflicted upon us by those who were meant to love and protect us, or by the traumas of life. We may wear our outside accomplishments well—nice make-up and outfit, a good career, a decent place to live. Yet, we still struggle with finding true contentment because we wonder if we are worthy of being loved or can trust that others will not hurt or betray us again.

Self-worth

Many women, even in their 40s, 50s, 60s, and beyond, still do not feel completely anchored in a true, deep, and undeniable sense of their worth, or are living lives full of protective boundaries they believe keep them emotionally safe, but ultimately, are robbing them of an ability to be meaningfully connected with others. This is one of the most painful aspects of my work: feeling a deep desire to pour validation into these female vessels but knowing that my contribution to their journey is but a drop in the bucket of what needs to happen for someone to truly take ownership of their place in this world. I sometimes feel like screaming, "You are so glorious! Such an incredible and intricate being, a goddess in your own right. Can you not see or feel that?" But I refrain and instead, gently take her by the hand and try to lead her down the road of personal ownership to begin filling herself with self-love, one daily ritual at a time.

For Eloise and countless other women who have not experienced a loving and nurturing childhood, or safe and trusting adult connections, it is often overwhelming to face the possibility that something can shift and change in their relationships. Many times, there is an imbalance in their current connections with others, where they are the strivers, over-extenders, and pleasers. These understandable strategies are an attempt to garner the approval, acceptance, and validation from their adult relationships that they never got from their childhood ones. Unfortunately, those drawn to such women offering boundless giving are sometimes scarred in their own right and seek to dominate, control, and eventually, even punish the tender hearts that offered themselves so willingly at first.

Eventually, the lopsided nature of these relationships begins to manifest itself in insidious ways. Under the constant stress of domineering relationships, I have seen women become physically and emotionally ill, withdraw from pursuing things that used to please them, and shrink down into a diminished version of themselves to survive. It is my life's mission to help women find their way back to a version of themselves that honors their uniqueness and allows them to fulfill their destiny. I truly feel that it is NEVER TOO LATE, no matter what someone has gone through, to commit to a different, enhanced way of being.

This doesn't just magically happen with enough psychotherapy. Rather, it is a daily practice of living with intention, being fully aware that each action we take has the potential to grow or diminish aspects of ourselves. No matter what I may deeply want for a client, she will have to want to change, for change to happen in her life.

Relationships

The work of deepening our connection with those currently in our lives, or reaching out to connect with others, takes work. In some cases, it may mean choosing to distance ourselves from those who are not honoring or respecting us. This is a very difficult and often very painful realization, and a decision fraught with intense emotions, such as fear and uncertainty. Many of us find ourselves in certain relationships that are just not supporting our emotional and physical health and are often damaging to us. There are many reasons why we choose to remain connected: financial, societal, and personal, like avoiding feeling lonely, but often, this decision comes at a price.

If you find yourself in a relationship that is unsafe, hurtful, or damaging, please seek local help or guidance to explore your options. But if distancing yourself from a toxic connection is feasible, you owe it to yourself to explore both why you would stay and what would potentially change if you left. Be honest with yourself about how interacting with someone is impacting your soul health. You may begin to discover truths that initially seemed insignificant but now have grown into a suffocating reality that is poisoning your life and potential for fulfilling your unique destiny.

Although Eloise initially continued to struggle with finding her true voice in her relationships, by choosing to live each day with mindful ritual and intention, she began to embrace each new day with a renewed sense of possibility, rather than dread. From taking an extra 5 minutes in the morning to engage in a gratitude practice of voicing out loud three things that she was grateful for to taking a moment to send a text message to a friend who was coping with a hospitalized parent, Eloise began to experience a sense of enhanced well-being and an improved ease and flow to her day. Now when she was sitting in traffic or waiting in a long line at the post office, she would take the time to take several calming and centering breaths in and out her nose, feeling her parasympathetic nervous system reboot, washing away her stress hormones. She then would find herself able to experience greater compassion and empathy for the people in line with her and for the workers fervently trying to take care of postal business.

Eloise felt the tremendous transformative potential of shifting from her previous rushed and disconnected way of interacting with the world, to a more meaningful and purposeful mode of existence. This awareness of her ability to access peace, ease, and connection with just a simple, yet intentional shift towards peace within herself was such a powerful and life-affirming realization that it began to build a foundation of healing. This eventually enabled her to cultivate deeper self-love and a true appreciation of her potential for change in other aspects of her life. The transformation I witnessed in Eloise brought such joy to my heart. I knew then that the third task of "Still standing, now what?" would come with greater ease for her.

The final part of our journey was based on the concept of deepening Eloise's understanding of her gifts and talents, and how they could be used to give back to the world. At first, this was very challenging because she was good at minimizing positive or worthy aspects of herself or would come up with myriad excuses for why she could not participate in the various opportunities we would brainstorm together.

Initially, we discovered that fear, still rooted in childhood experiences of not being accepted, was still gripping her sense of her inherent value and worth, essentially smothering any potential of her adult self to feel confident enough to embark upon novel social situations. We spent time discussing how, for so many years of raising her children and beyond, she had essentially put herself on hold.

This overdoing for those closest to her had been her attempt to be a loving and giving mother and wife, but ironically, had left her feeling depleted and resentful. There was no doubt that she loved her family and would always try to be there for them, but the process of starting to build up her physical and emotional vitality had created a possibility for change across other domains of her current life. Once that momentum had taken hold, Eloise began to embrace her potential for a different way of being.

Over time, Eloise's excuses softened, and she began to recognize the value of doing, no matter how small the gesture. We had often discussed her love of movies and thought that she might be able to give back by donating movies to the local women's shelter where they might provide a sense of comfort and inspiration to women who were working to rebuild their footing in life. I knew that unless Eloise felt deeply aligned with the proposed project, and it mattered to her, it would not serve the intended purpose: to deepen her sense of self-worth, efficacy, and purpose, no matter what life stage she was in. It wasn't until Eloise listened to that still, small voice inside that she was able to be present for herself and to proceed with a strong sense of intention and purpose for her life.

In all of this exploration of "Still standing, now what?" we are not aiming to arrive at some particular destination, but rather, we are working towards being kinder, gentler, and more open to what is available to all of us, all around us, one day at a time. I think of it as being more present in our daily lives to be able to see, feel, and experience the infinite potential of each day, with its beautiful and not so wonderful moments. I think the question of "Still standing, now what?" needs to be answered for each one of us with a deep examination of how we choose to be in each day that we are given on this Earth.

Are we choosing to live with gratitude or are we allowing the cluttered, worried thoughts to steal the joy out of even the most glorious of moments? I know, even for myself, that I have needed to train my mind, just as you would train your puppy to find the grace in interactions with difficult people, to lead with empathy, not retaliation, and to actively cultivate a sense of serenity in my daily routine, no matter what is going on around me. This is a choice, just like choosing what we are going to put on in the morning. The outcome is up to us.

I am here to help guide women, but ultimately, if I can connect them back to their inner compass of feminine intuition, then their voices will be heard. I am confident that they will take this precious moment and make something meaningful out of it. For it is in embracing each day with mindful intention that there is a possibility in even the tiniest choice, that we can live fully, fiercely, and without regrets.

I want to live with such vitality and ferocity, don't you? It IS possible, and it begins with knowing that you are worthy of finding the unique strength and beauty of your feminine power. Go forth and reclaim your life. I am encouraging and cheering you on!

CHAPTER 14 TIPS

1. Your midlife story is waiting to be written. Who will you choose to be and what will you choose to do?

2. All of us are walking wounded, but it is what we decide to believe about our potential to change the trajectory of our life is what ultimately allows us to align with our inner voice and live the life we are meant to live.

3. Aim to surround yourself with people who inspire you to be a better person or to lead a more fulfilling life. As we outgrow relationships and decide to leave them behind, we create the space for new people and new experiences to enrich our lives.

4. Identify one or two things you want more of in life and take one new step each day to try to make those wishes a new reality.

5. Even when we are struggling, there is always at least one thing we can be grateful for. Please make it a habit to start your day expressing gratitude for something in your life.

6. The possibility to change is within each one of us. We have to want it badly enough. Still standing? Then you have it in you to start today to change the things that are preventing you from living your best life. No one knows the beauty and potential inside of you until you allow it to shine, fully illuminating the world.

For attractive lips, speak words of kindness.

For lovely eyes, seek out the good in people.

For a slim figure, share your food with the hungry.

For beautiful hair, let a child run their fingers through it once a day.

For poise, walk with the knowledge that you never walk alone.

People, more than things, have to be restored, renewed, revived, reclaimed, and redeemed.

Remember, if you ever need a helping hand, you will find one at the end of each of your arms.

As you grow older, you will discover that you have two hands, one for helping yourself and the other for helping others.

SAM LEVENSON

References

1. Garber JR et al. Clinical practice guidelines for hypothyroidism in adults: Cosponsored by the American Association of Clinical Endocrinologists and the American Thyroid Association. Endocr Pract 2012 Nov/Dec; 18:988.

2. Sowers M et al. Thyroid stimulating hormone (TSH) concentrations and menopausal status in women at the mid-life: SWAN. Clin Endocrinol (Oxf) 2003 Mar; 58:340.

3. U.S. Preventive Services Task Force (USPSTF).Screening for thyroid disease: Recommendation statement. Ann Intern Med 2004 Jan 20; 140:125. (http://dx.doi.org/10.7326/0003-4819-140-2-200401200-00014)

4. Dr. Catherine Northrup/NAMI

5. www.health.harvard.edu/womens Harvard Health Publications Harvard Medical School Perimenopause: Rocky road to menopause.

You might also enjoy:

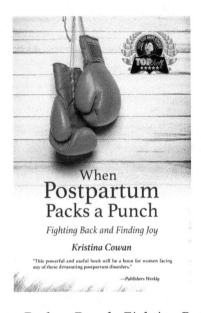

When Postpartum Packs a Punch: Fighting Back and Finding Joy
by Kristina Cowan

"This powerful and useful book will be a boon for women facing any of these devastating postpartum disorders."
—Publishers Weekly

When Postpartum Packs a Punch offers solace to mothers who have faced traumatic birth and perinatal mood disorders. Within the book is a chorus of different voices—parents, experts, and researchers—singing the same song: while the U.S. has made strides in caring for new mothers, we still have far to go. Stigma silences women, and blinds those on the sidelines. Stories of others' struggles are an antidote for stigma, because they let mothers know that they're not alone.

PraeclarusPress.com

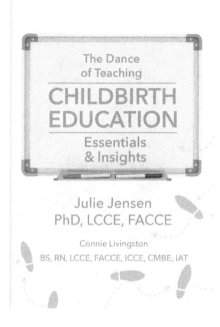

*The Dance of Teaching Childbirth Education: Essentials &
Insights*
by Julie Jensen

The Dance of Teaching Childbirth Education is a comprehensive book for childbirth educators and other perinatal practitioners that contains the practical essentials and insights in all areas of this wonderful field. Your journey is a dance of coordinating many moves to meet your needs and those of your learners. This book teaches you to incorporate evidence-based practices and create a curriculum to help you empower your participants and yourself.

PraeclarusPress.com

9 781946 665379